Who's making that noise?

Philip Hawthorn and Jenny Tyler
Illustrated by Stephen Cartwright

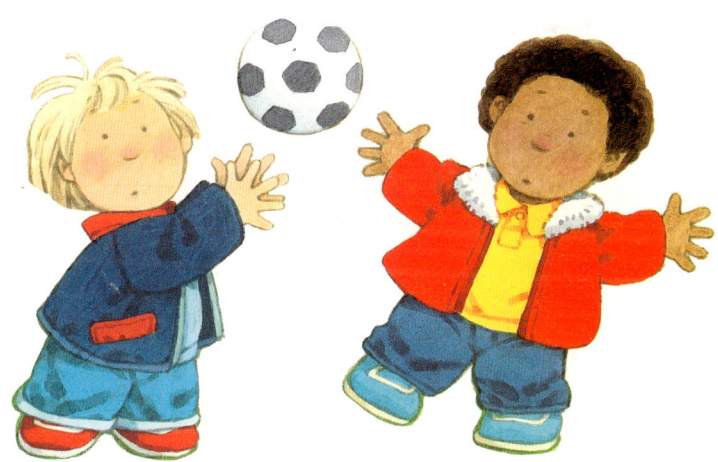

 There is a little yellow duck and a white mouse on every double page. Can you find them?

Who's making that noise?
Is it those noisy boys?

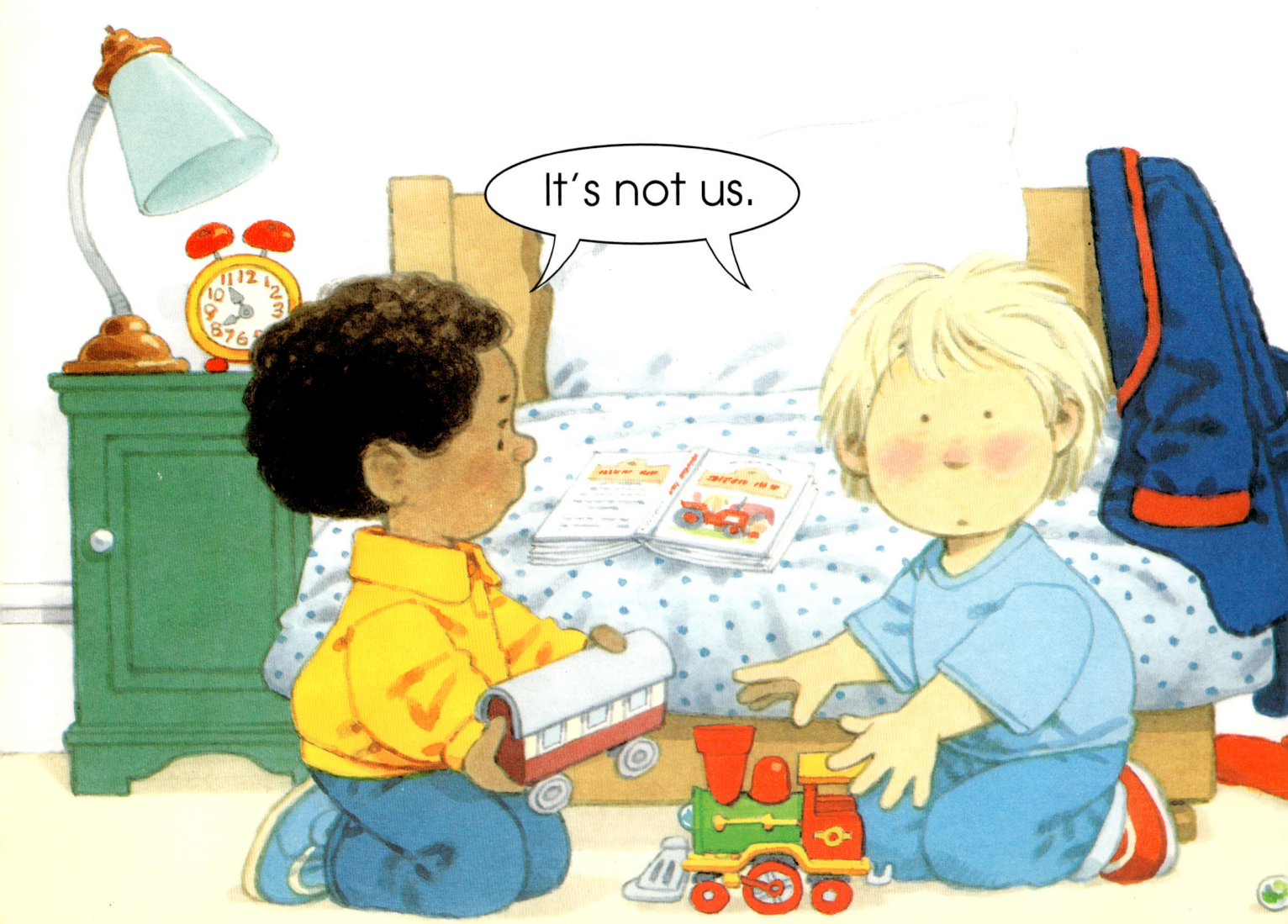

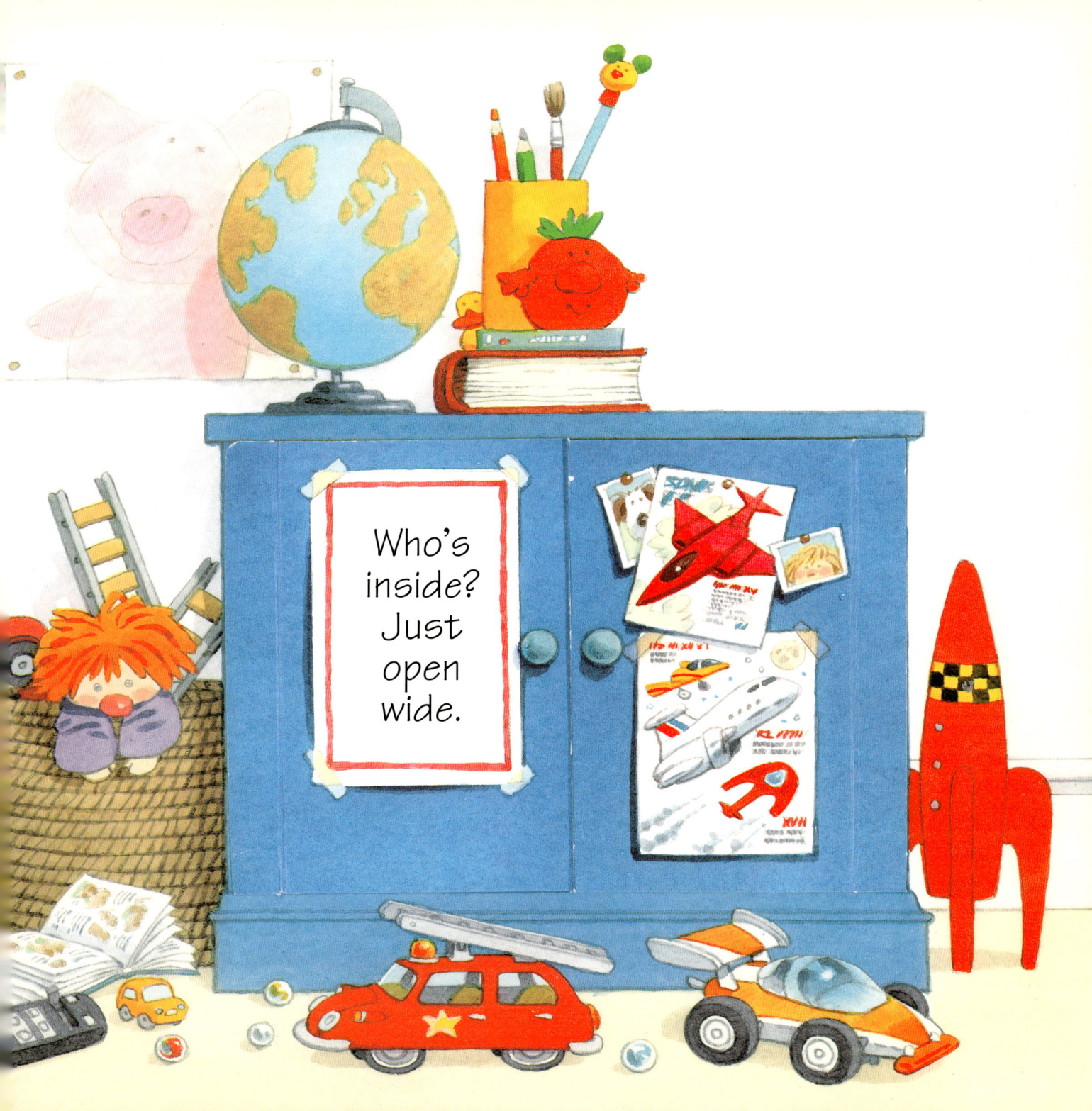

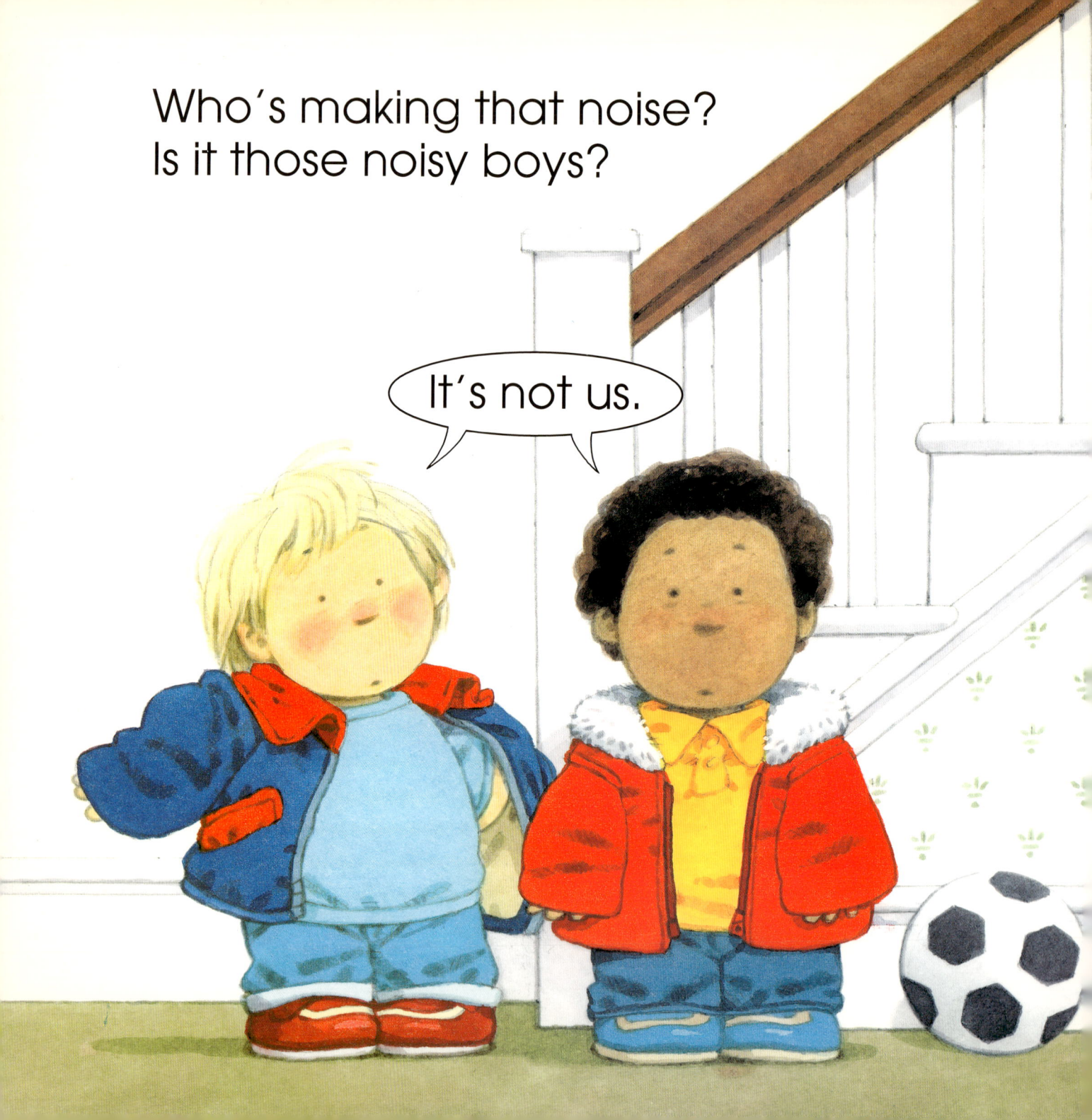

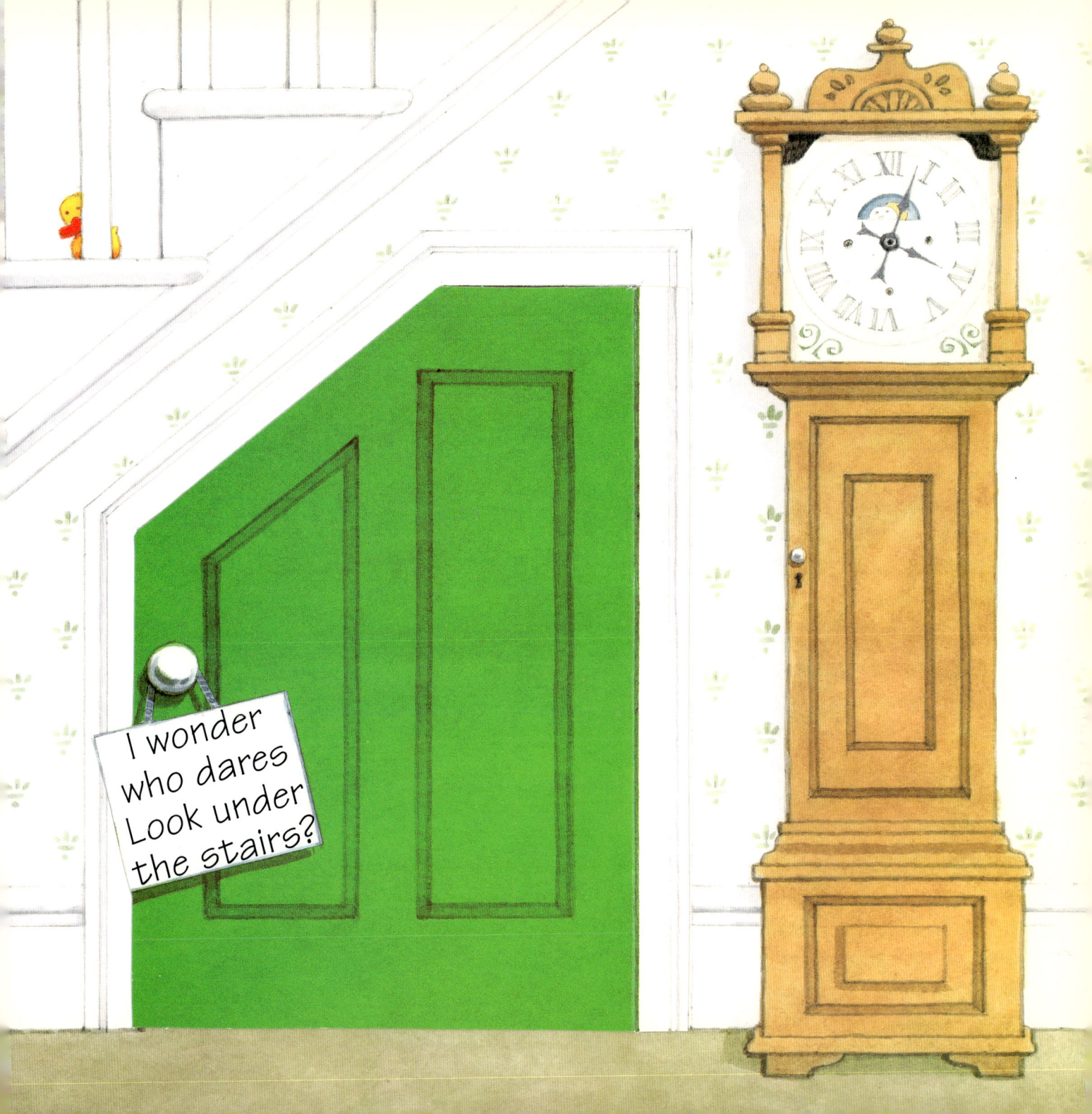

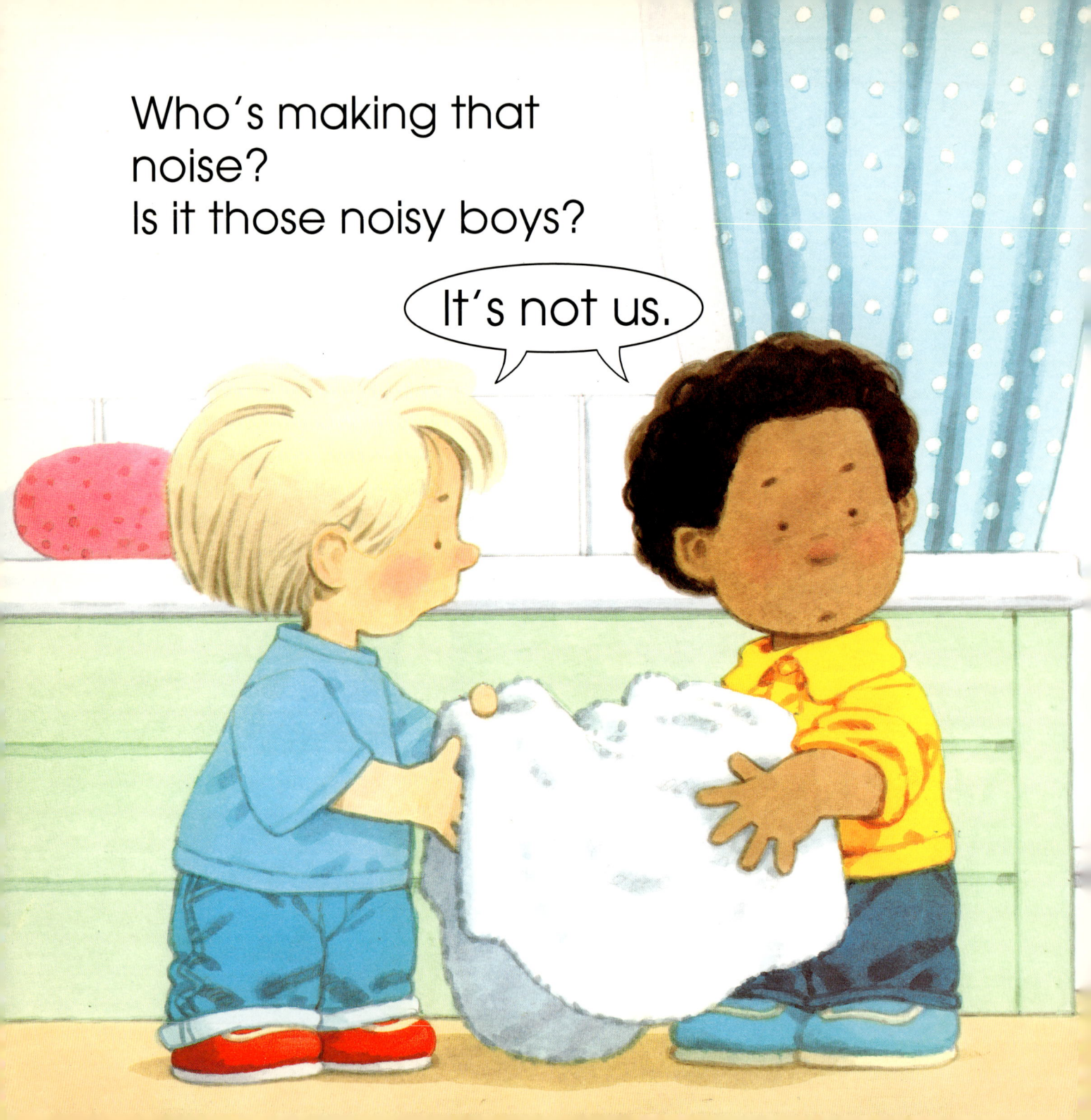

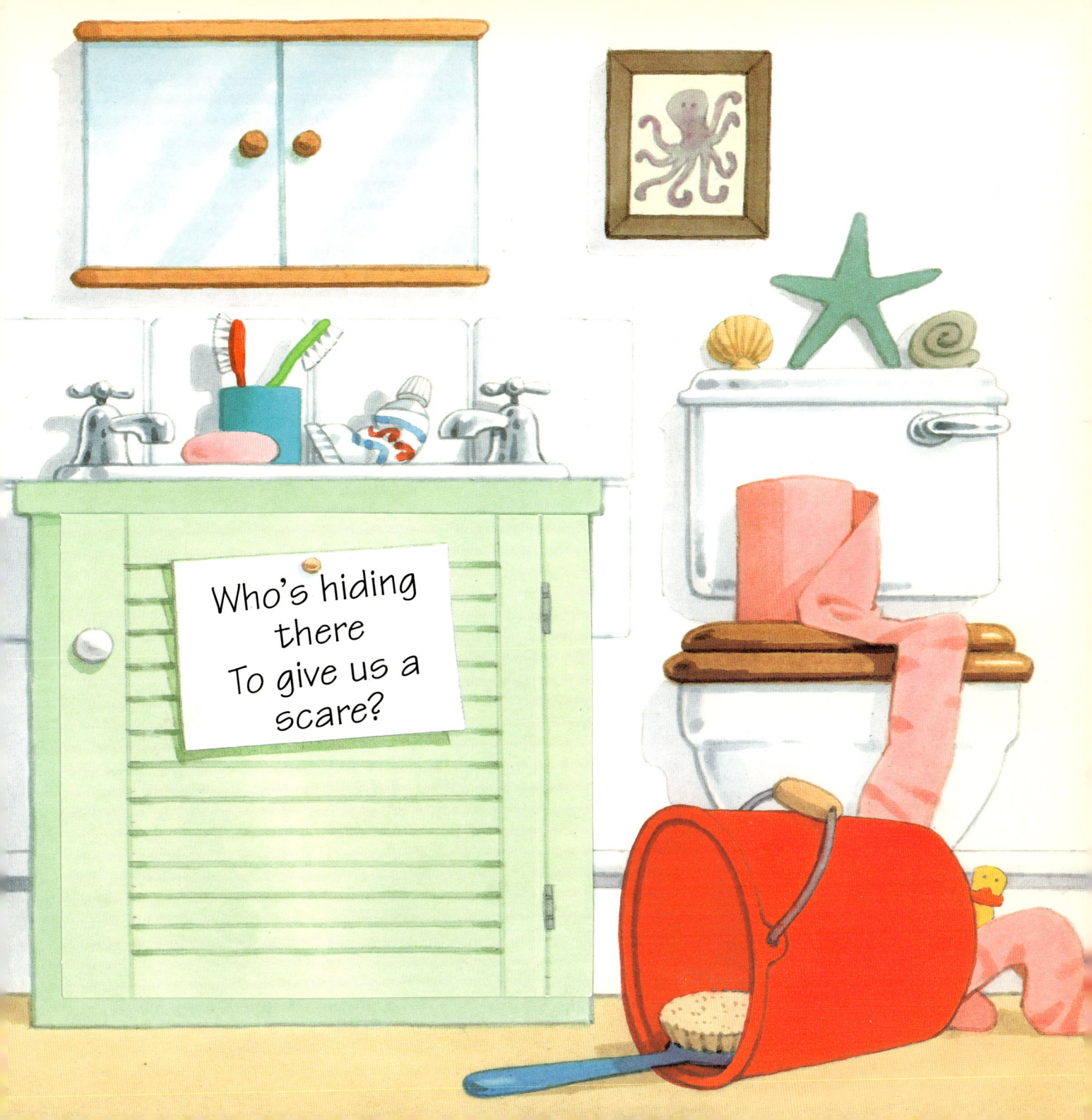

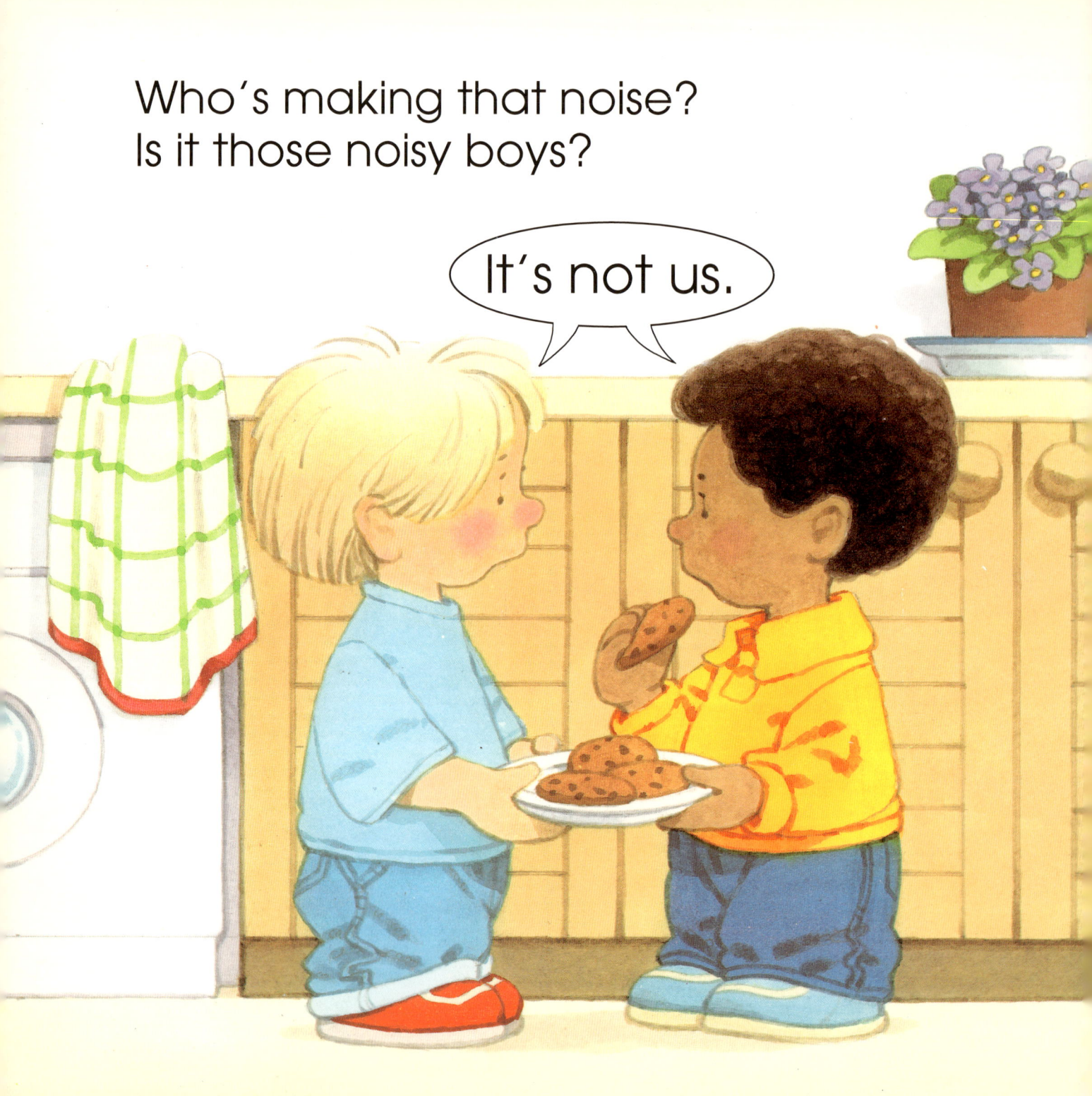

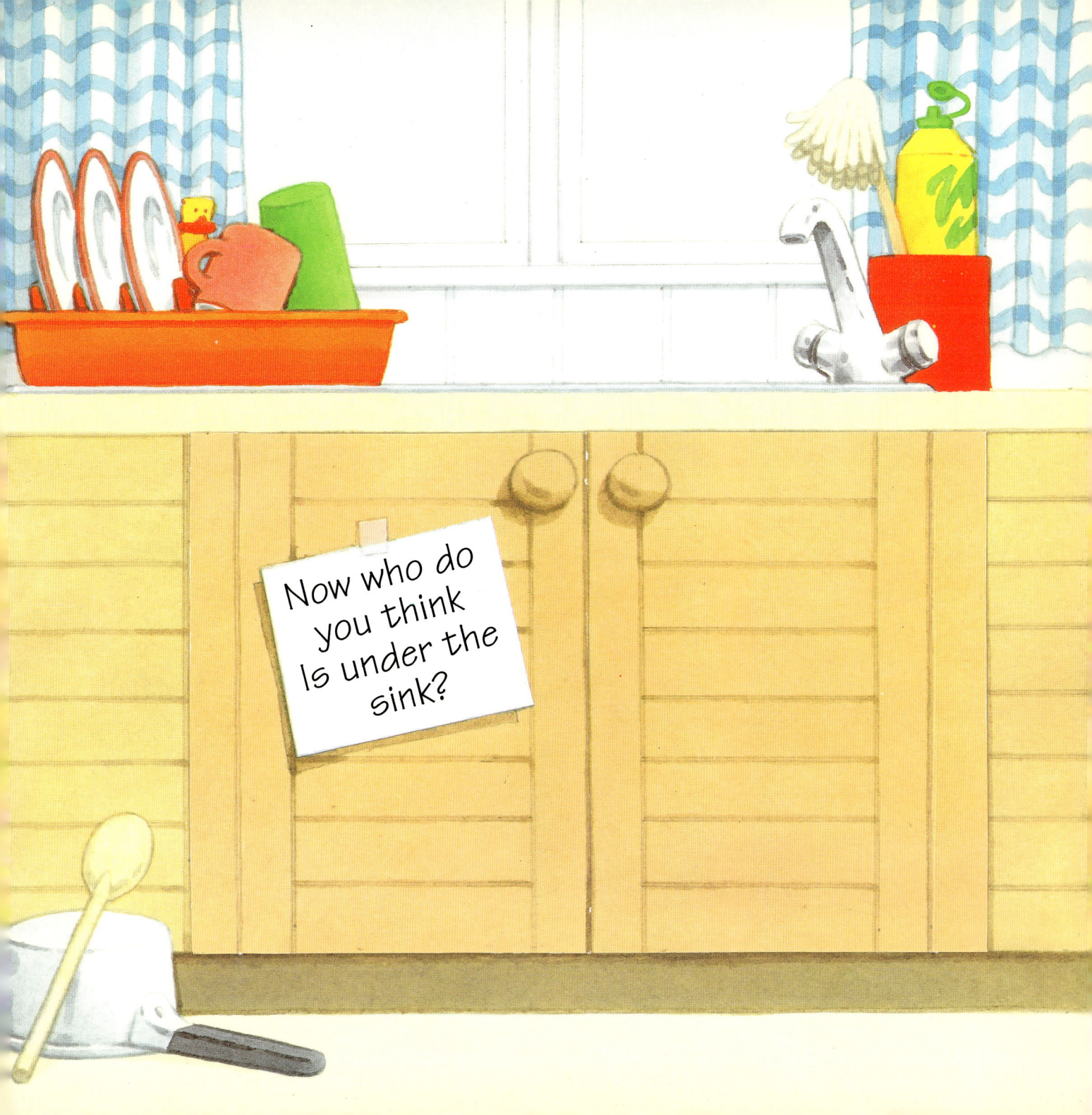

Who's making that noise?
Is it those noisy boys?

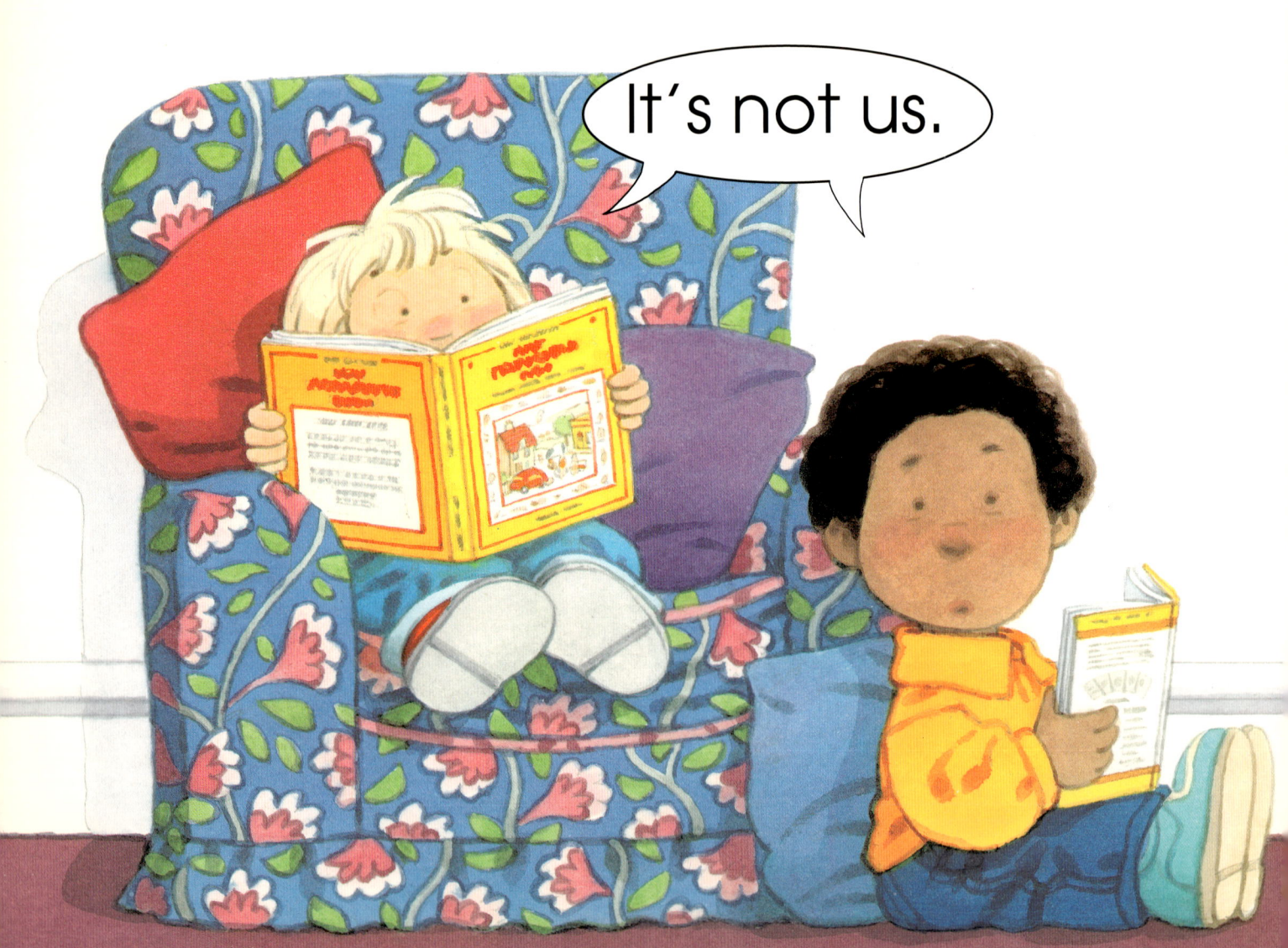

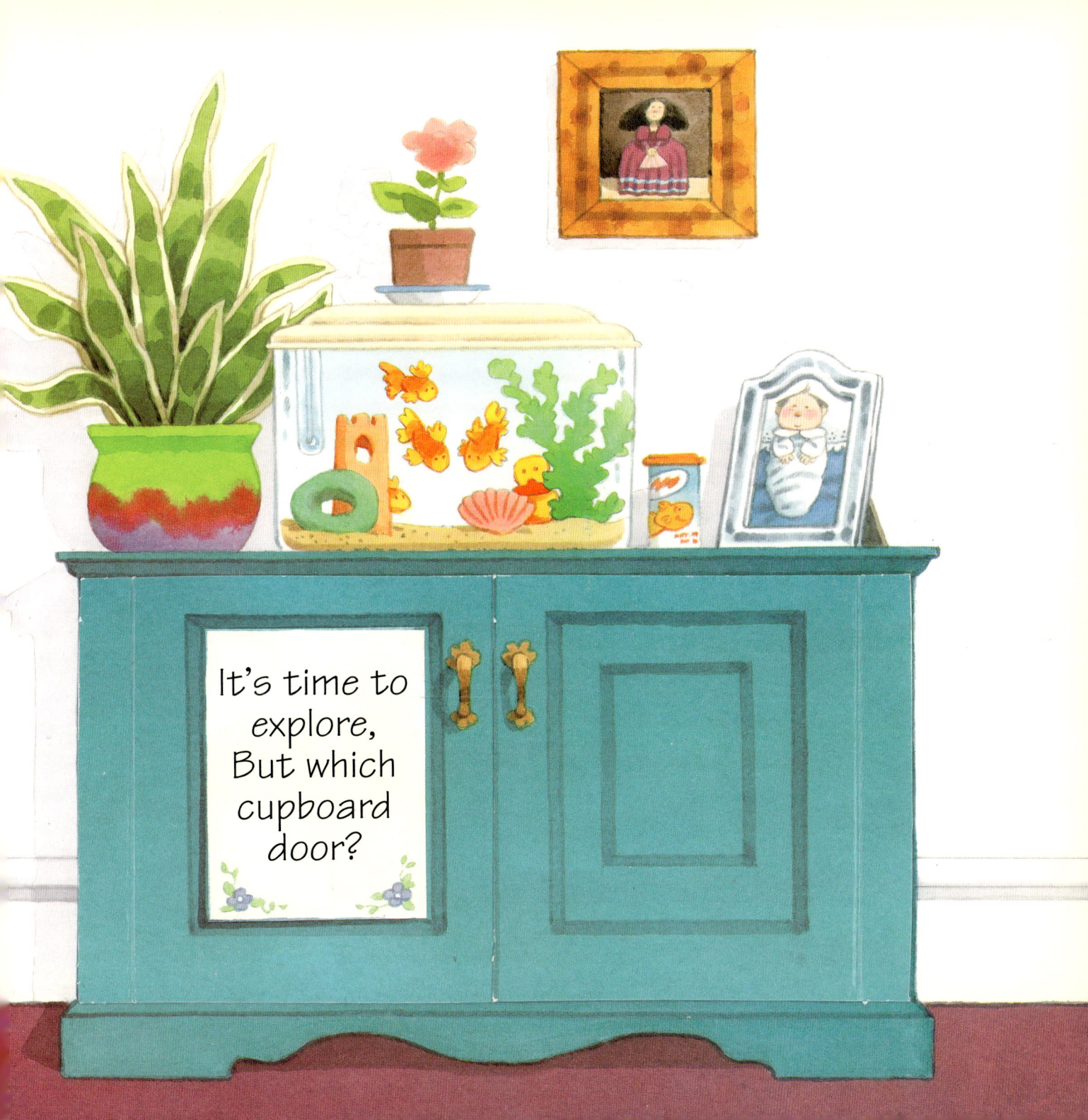

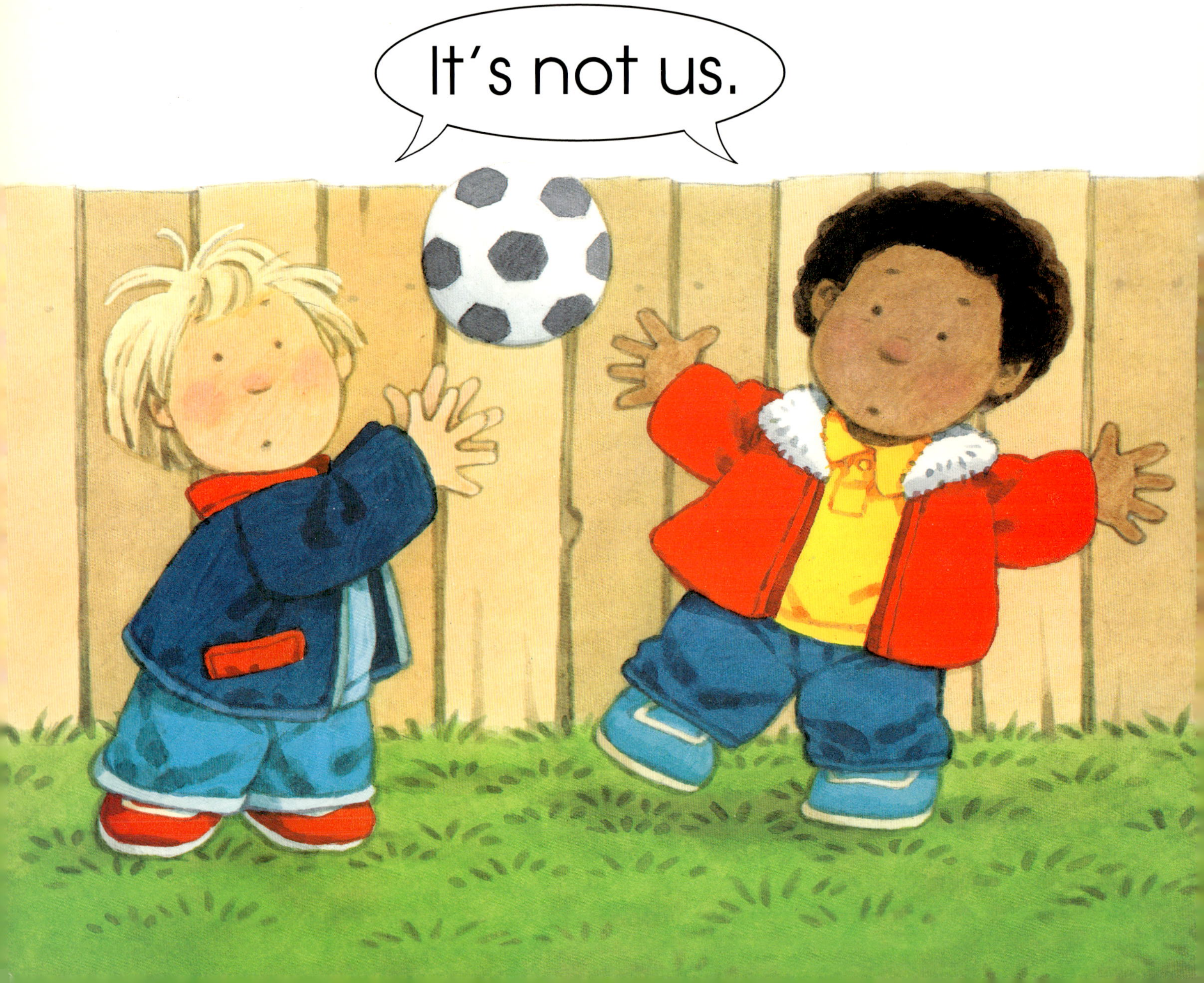

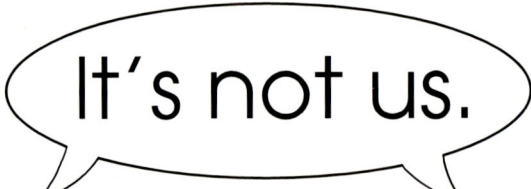

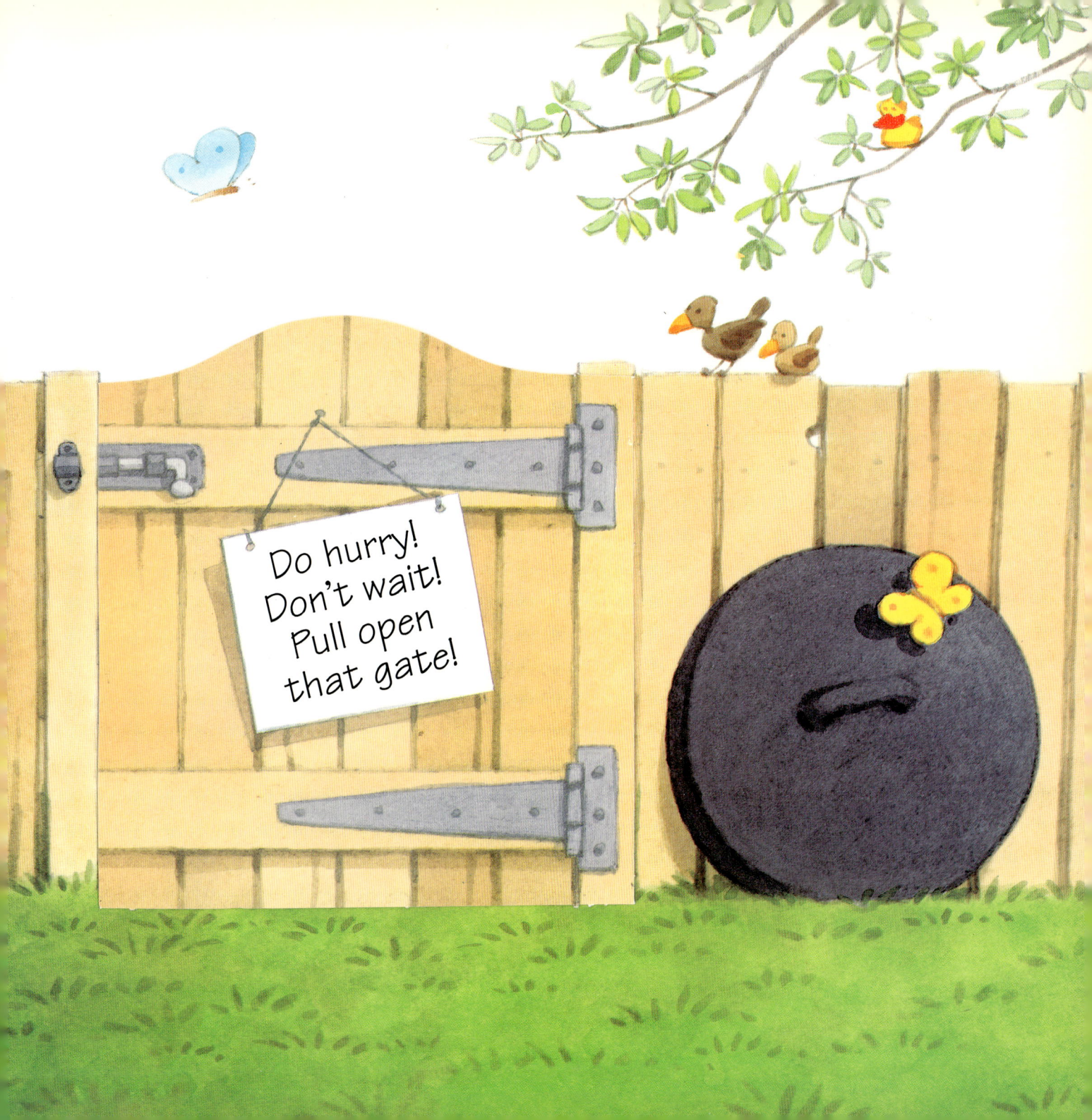

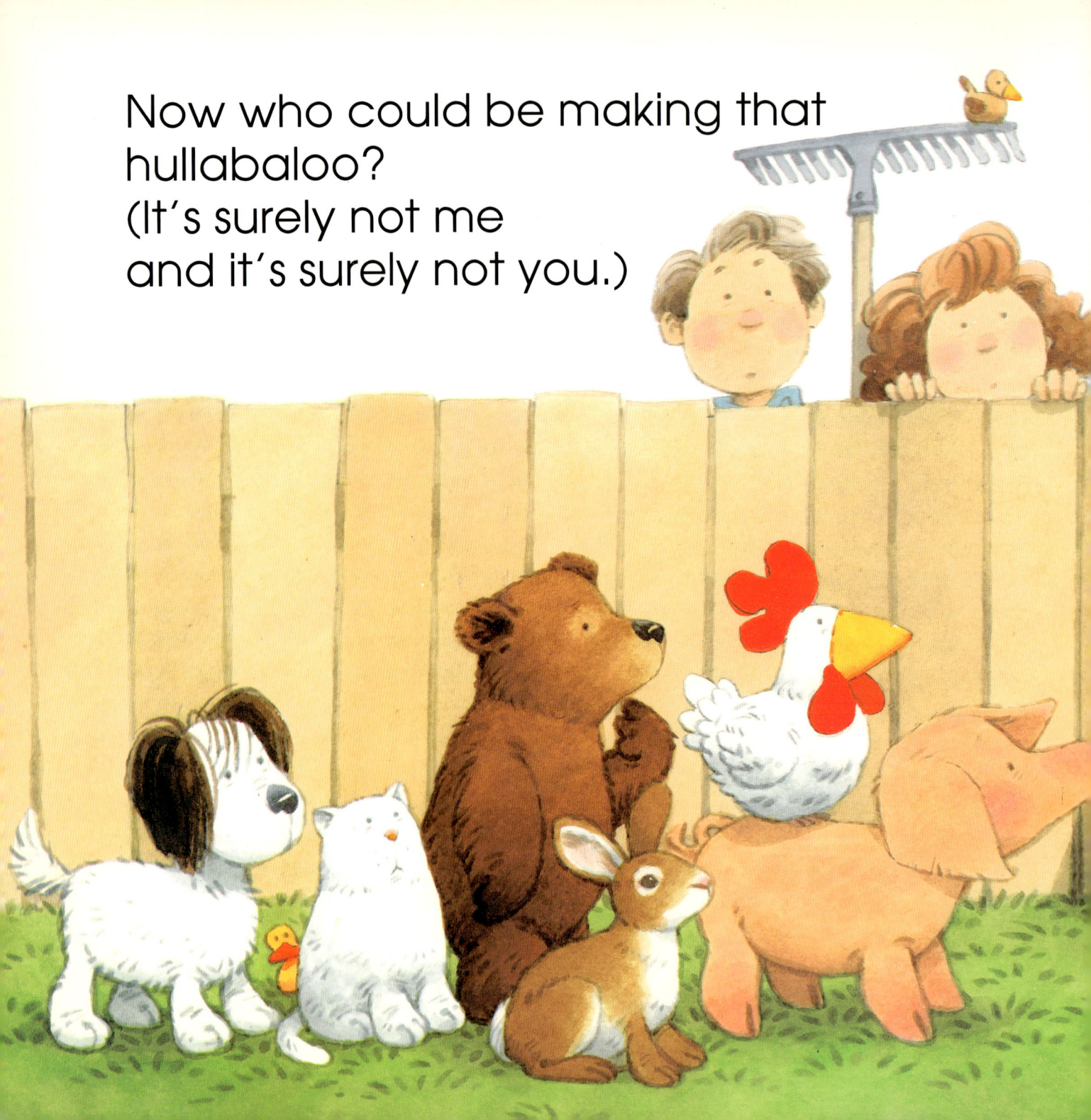
Now who could be making that hullabaloo?
(It's surely not me
and it's surely not you.)

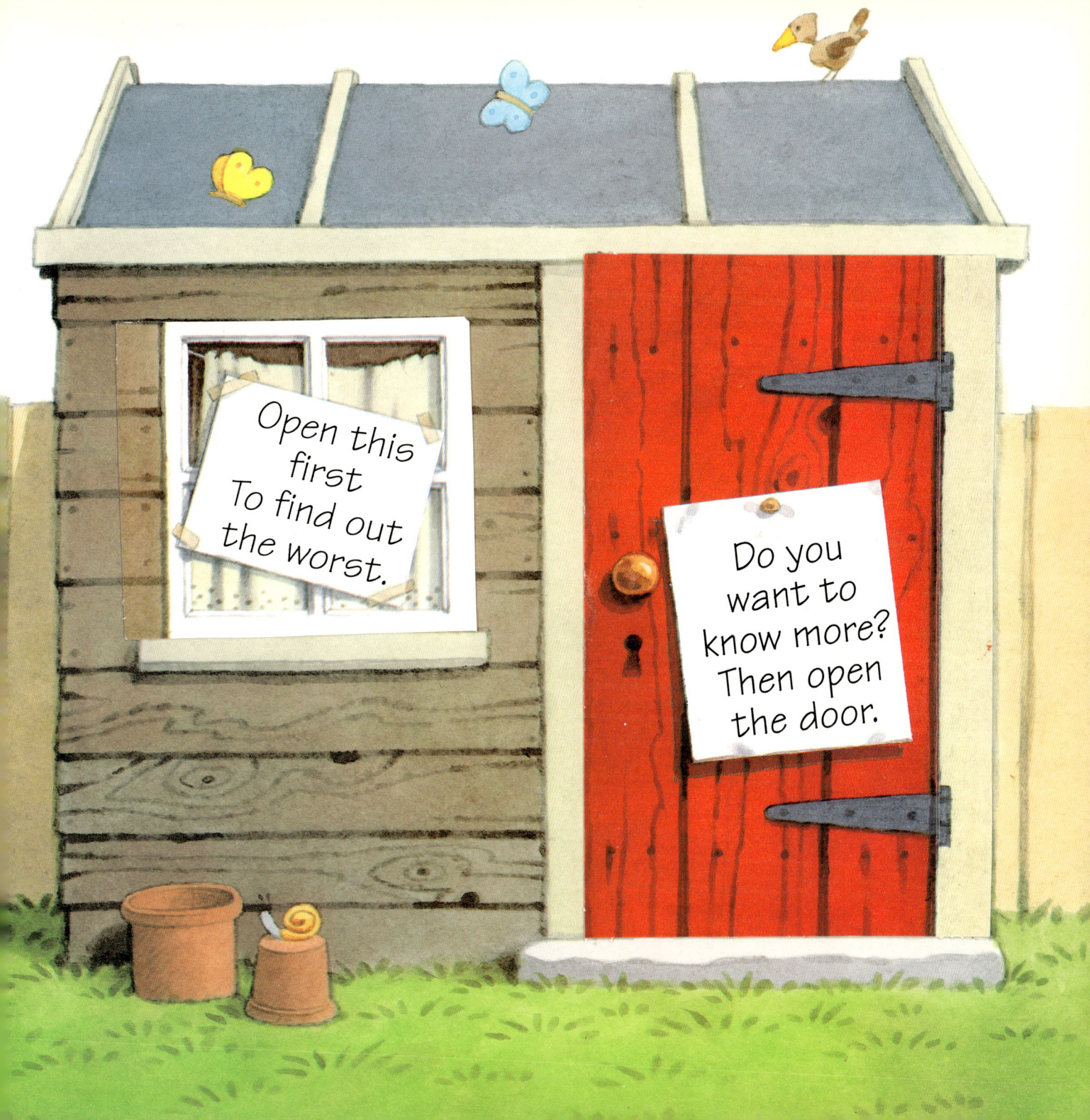

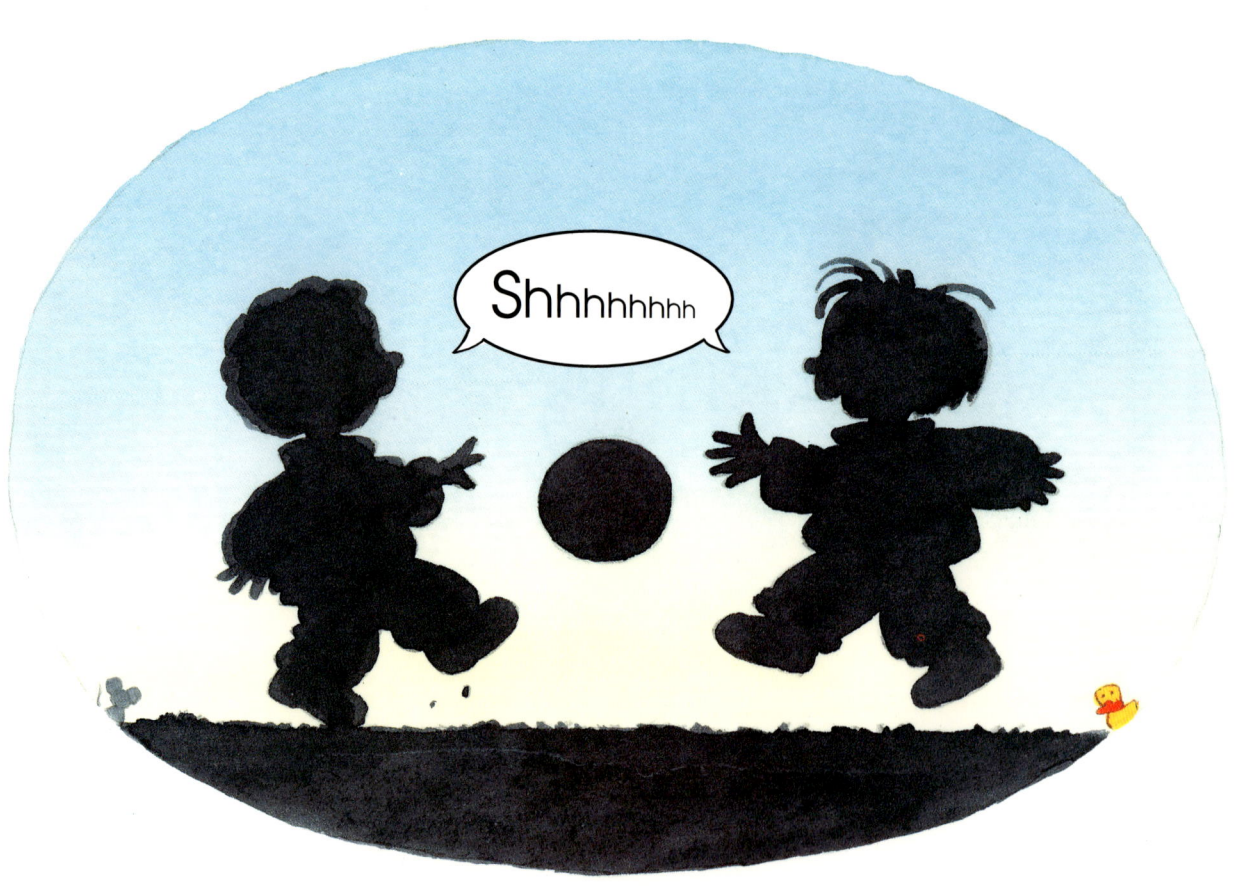

Who's making that smell?

Philip Hawthorn and Jenny Tyler
Illustrated by Stephen Cartwright

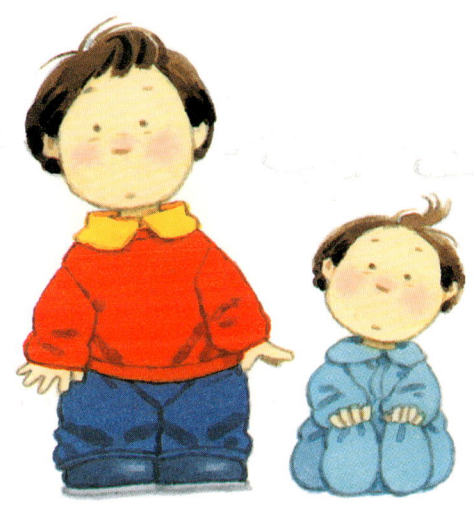

 There is a little yellow duck and a white mouse to look out for on every double page.

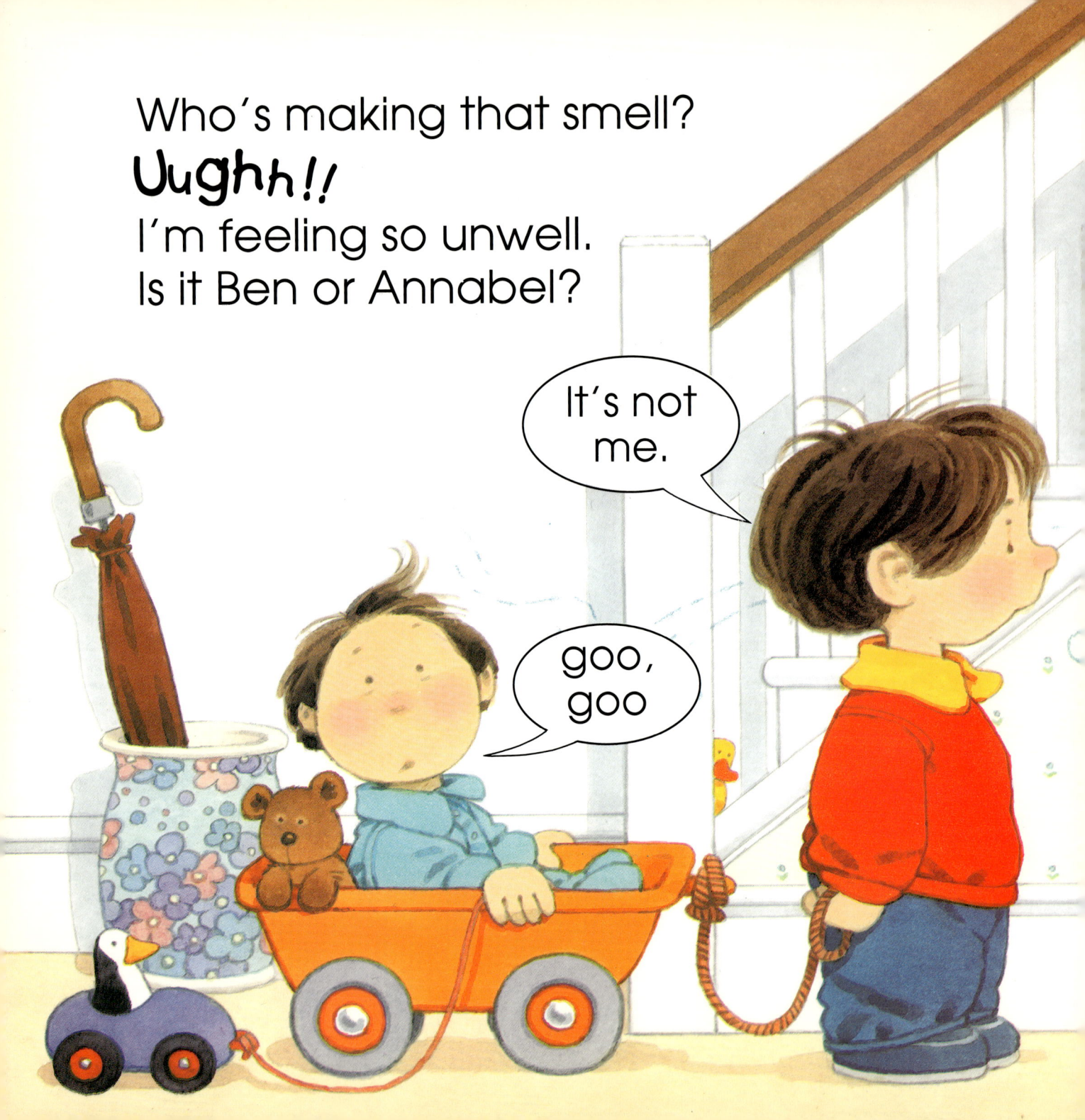

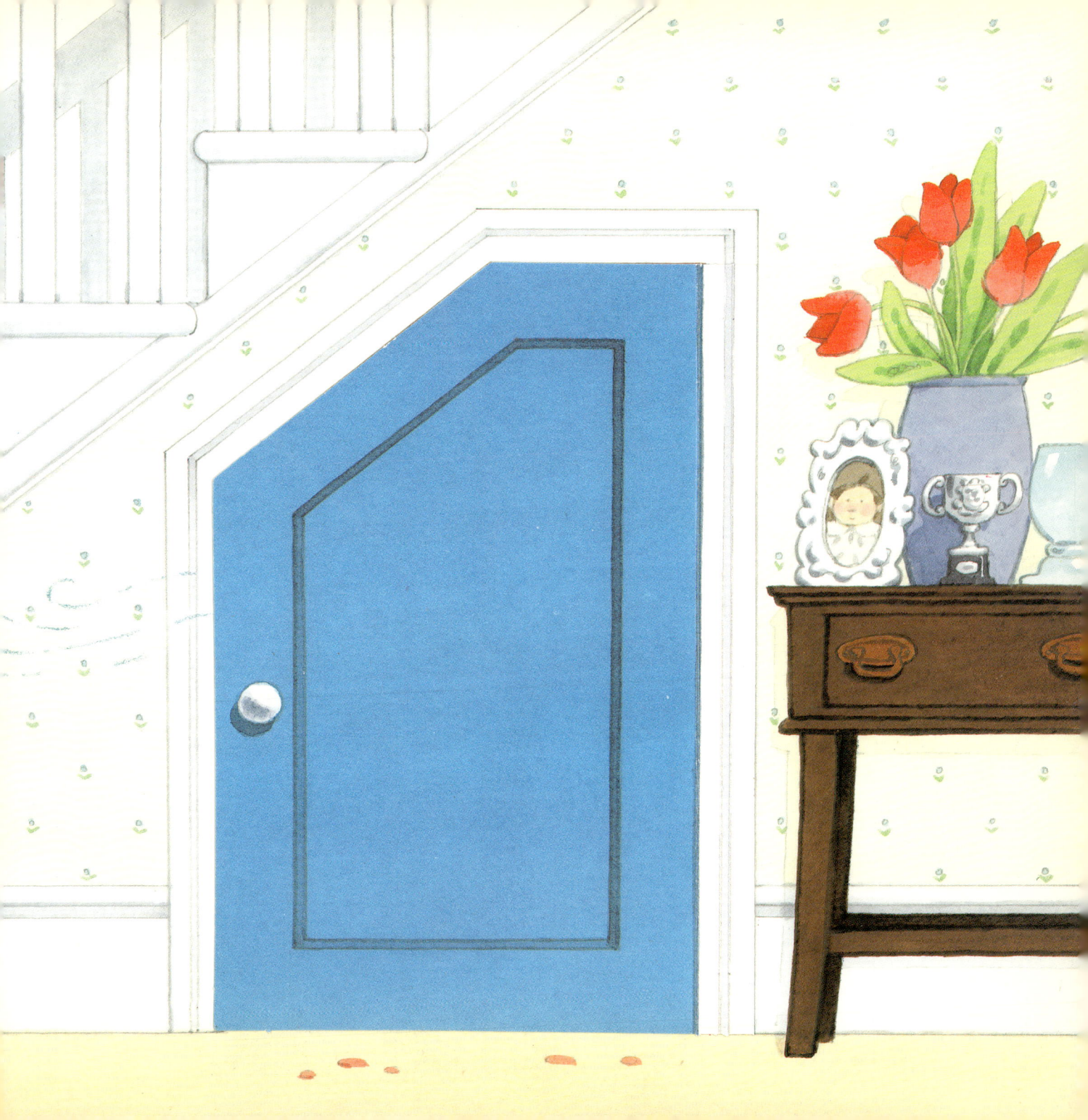

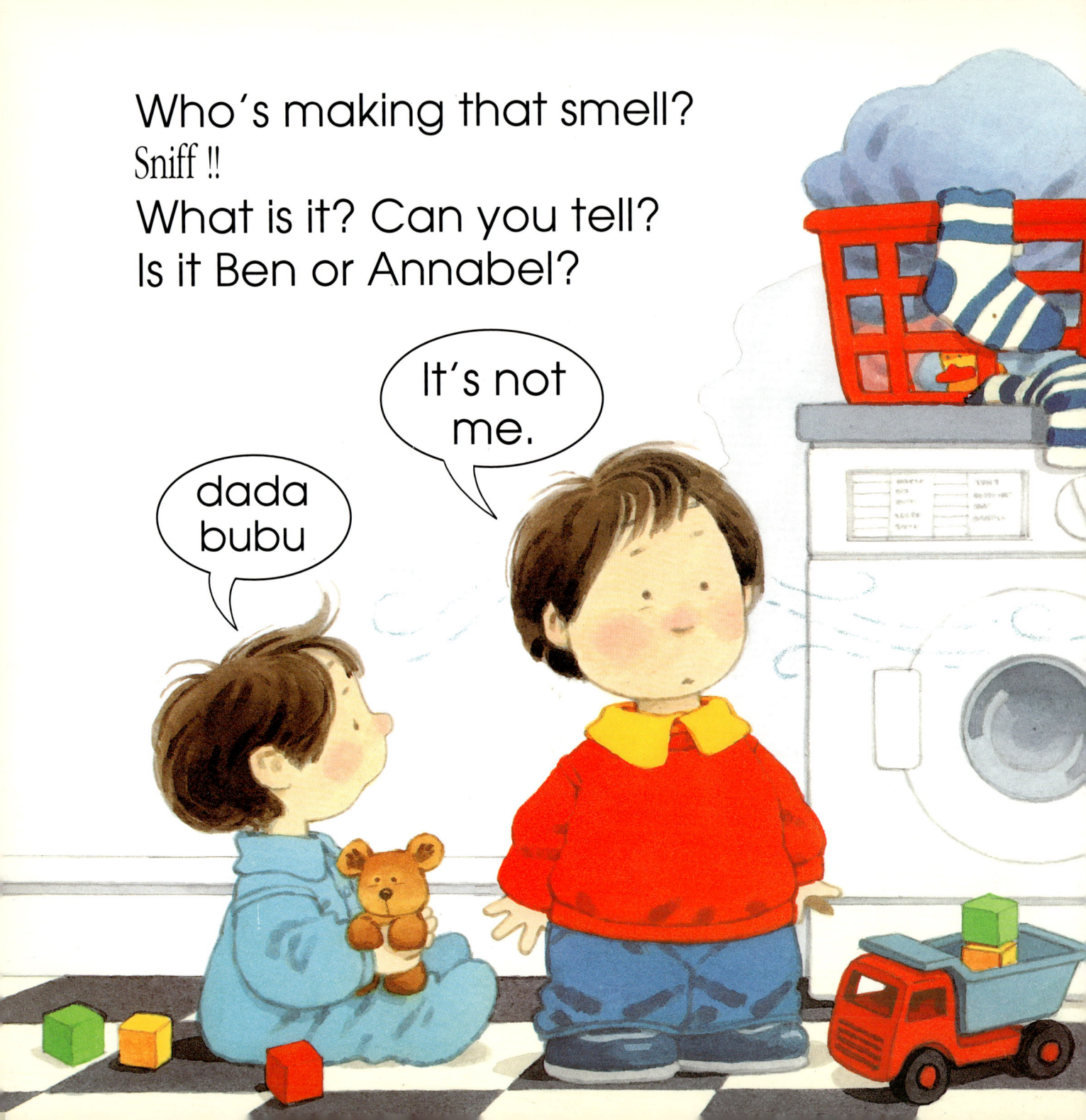

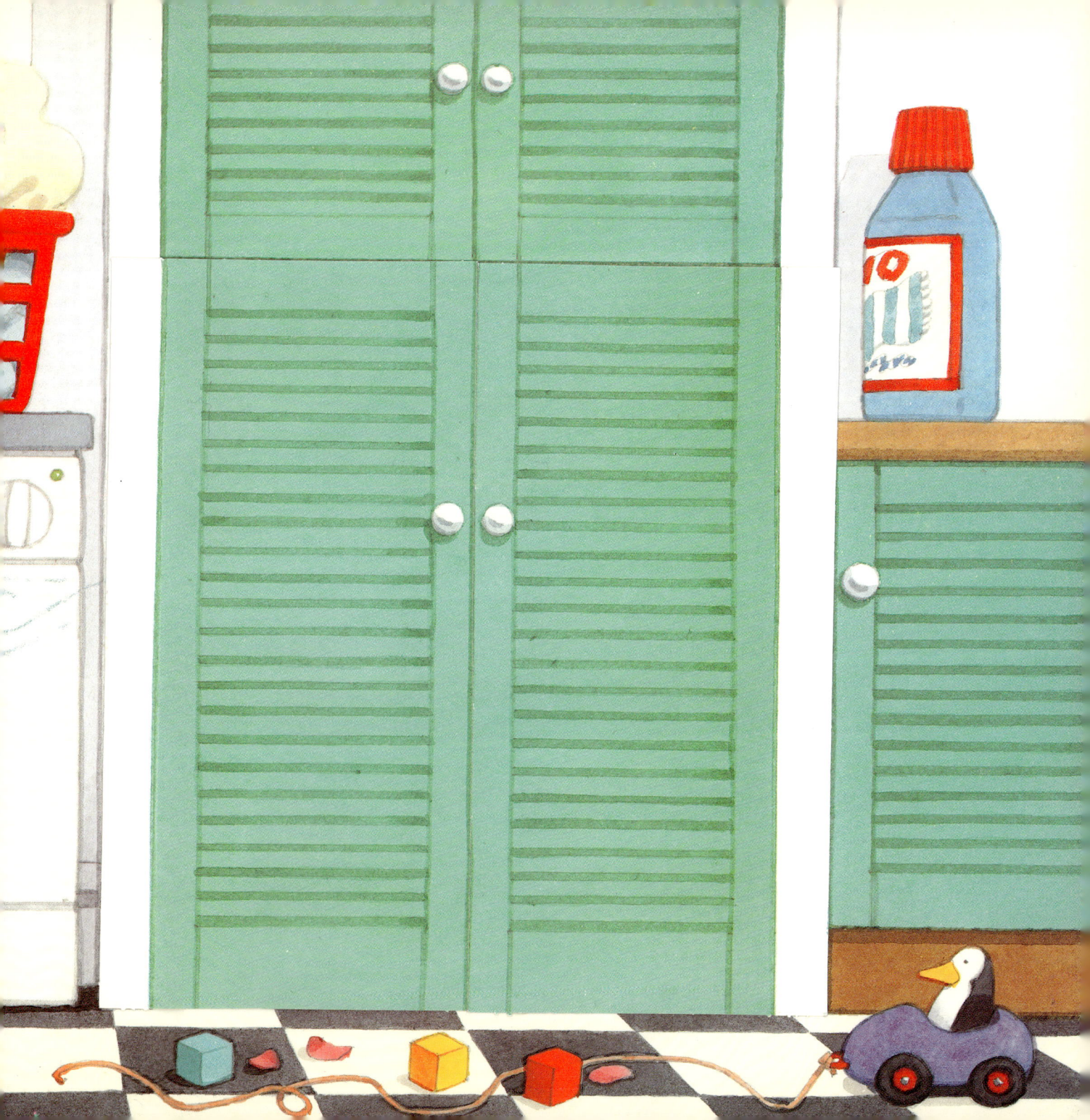

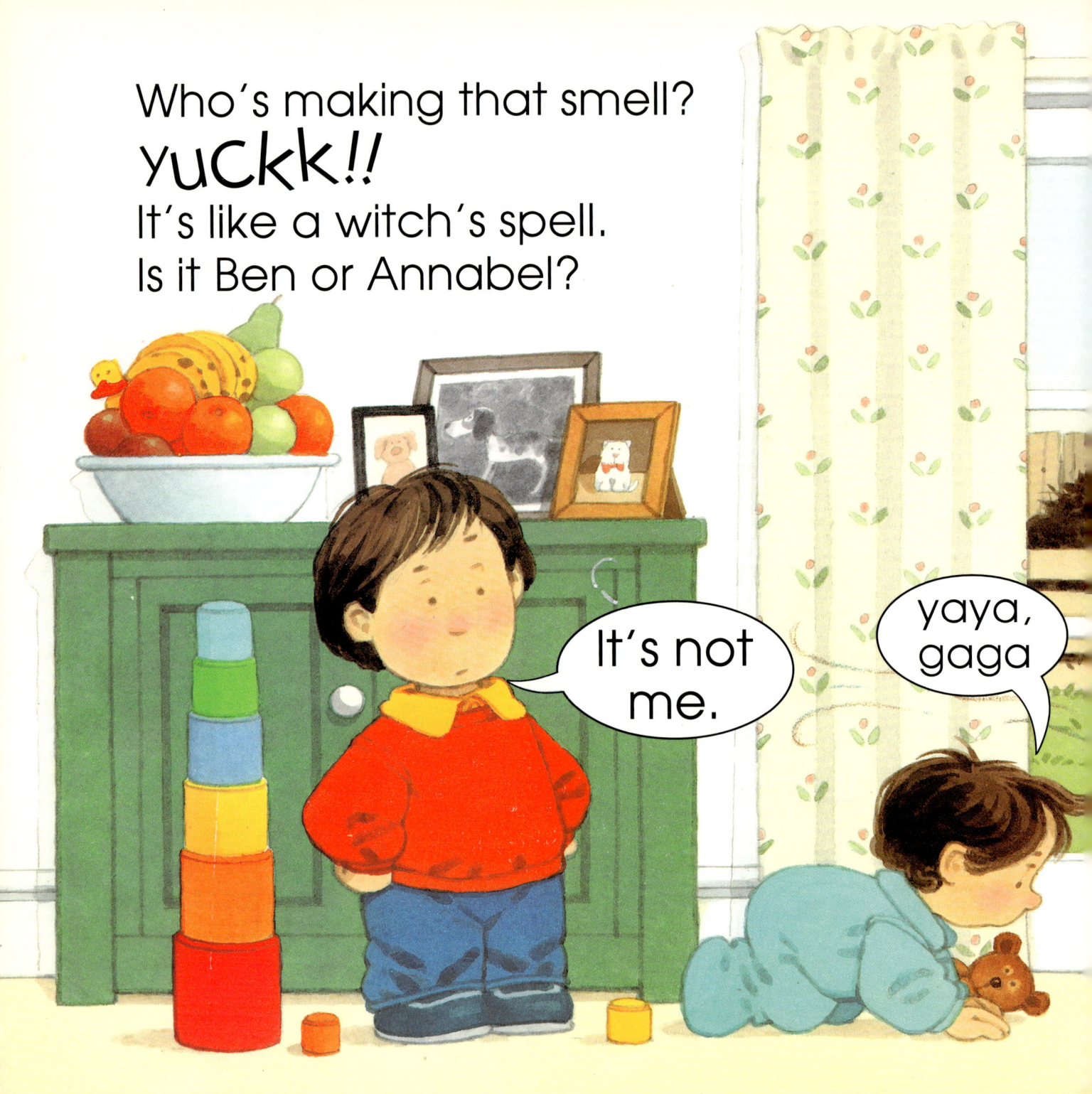

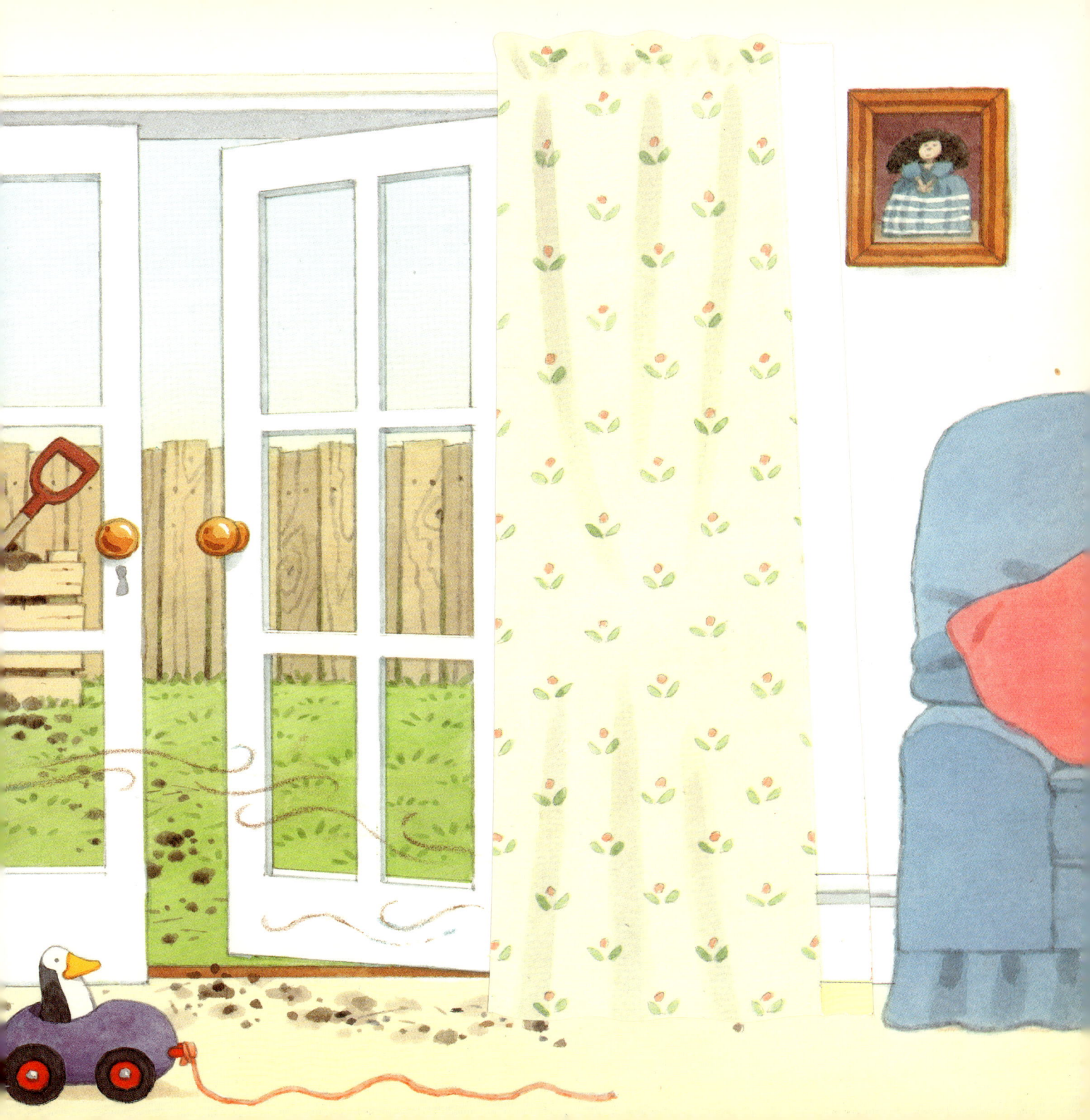

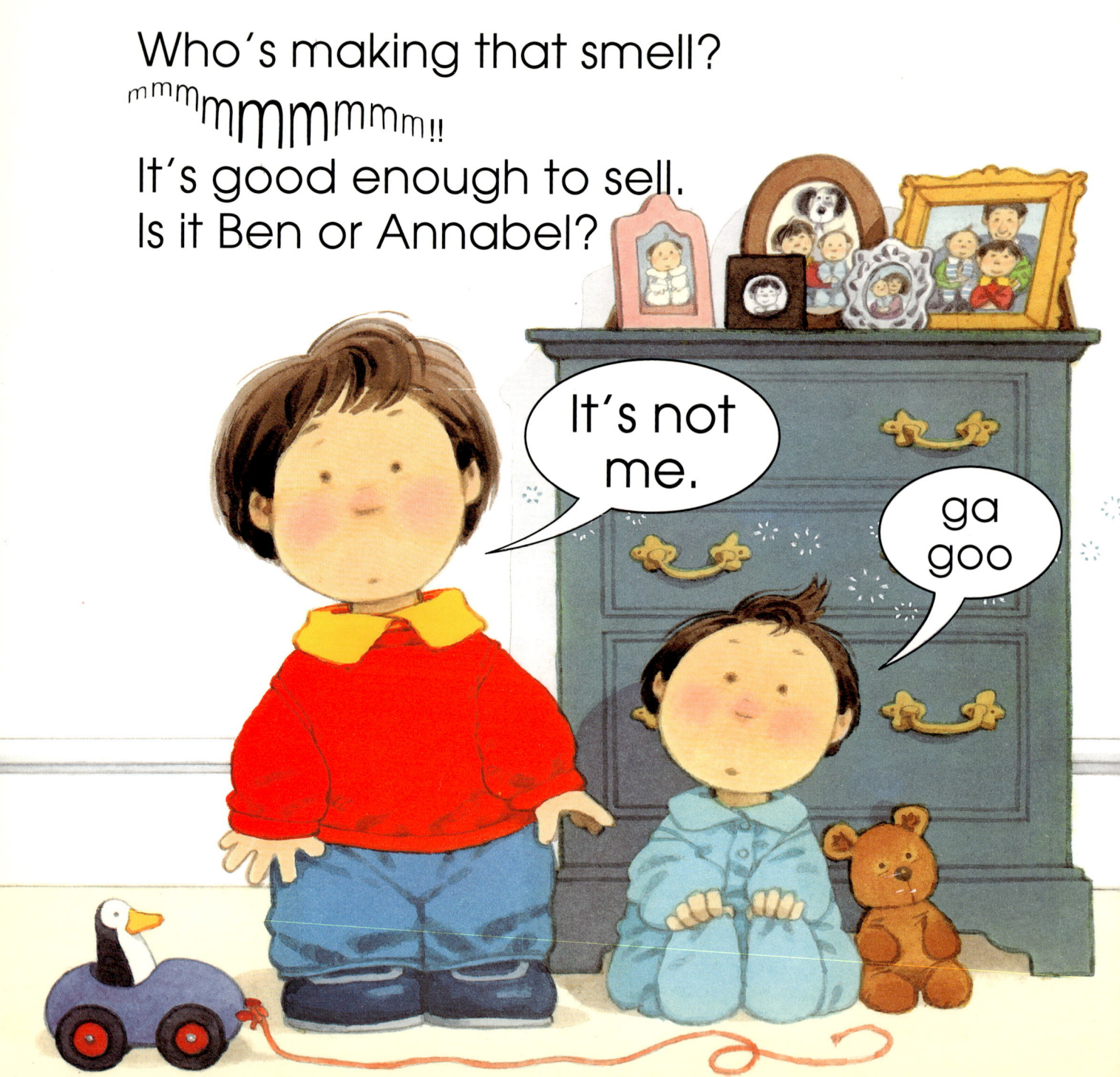

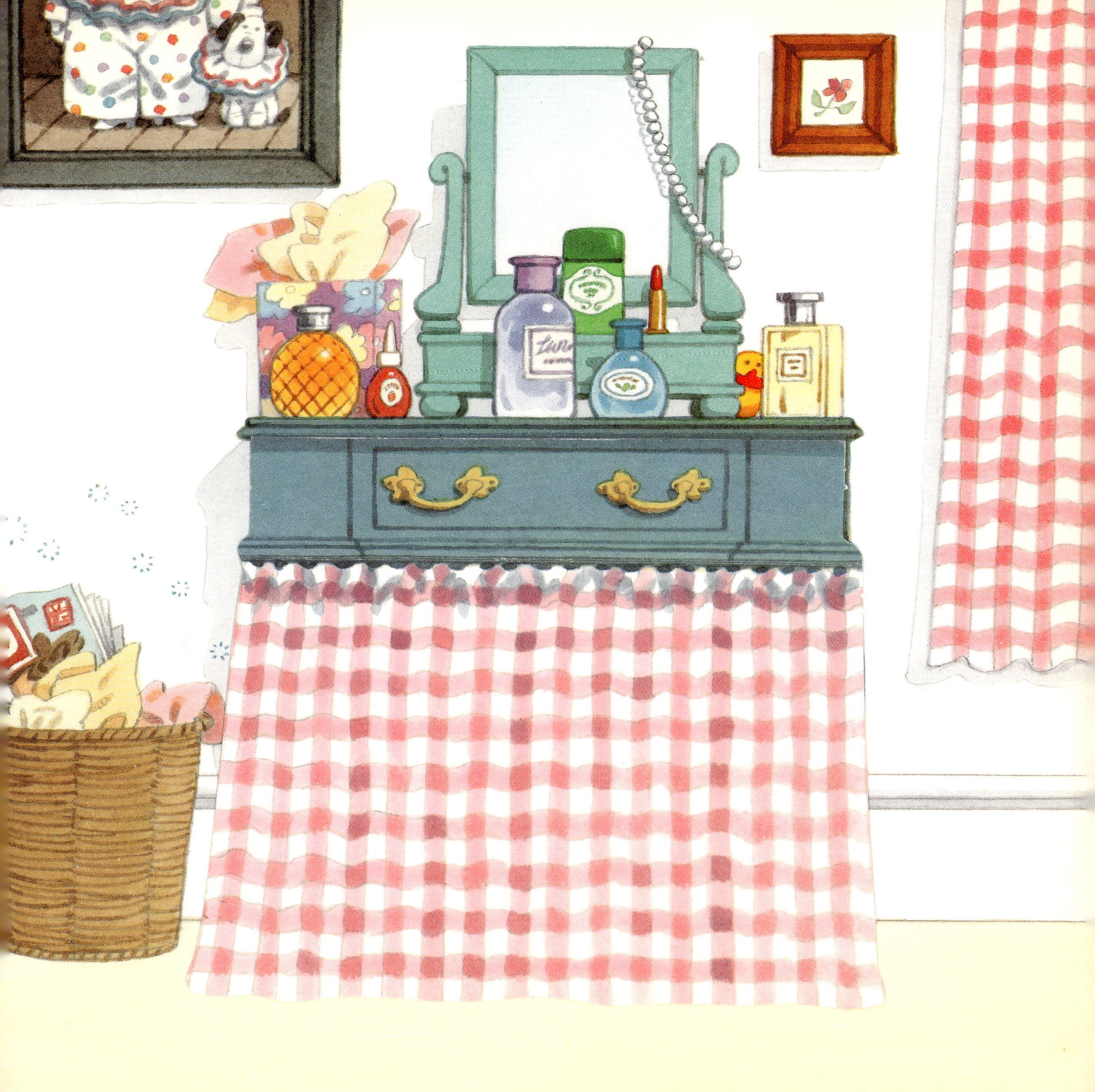

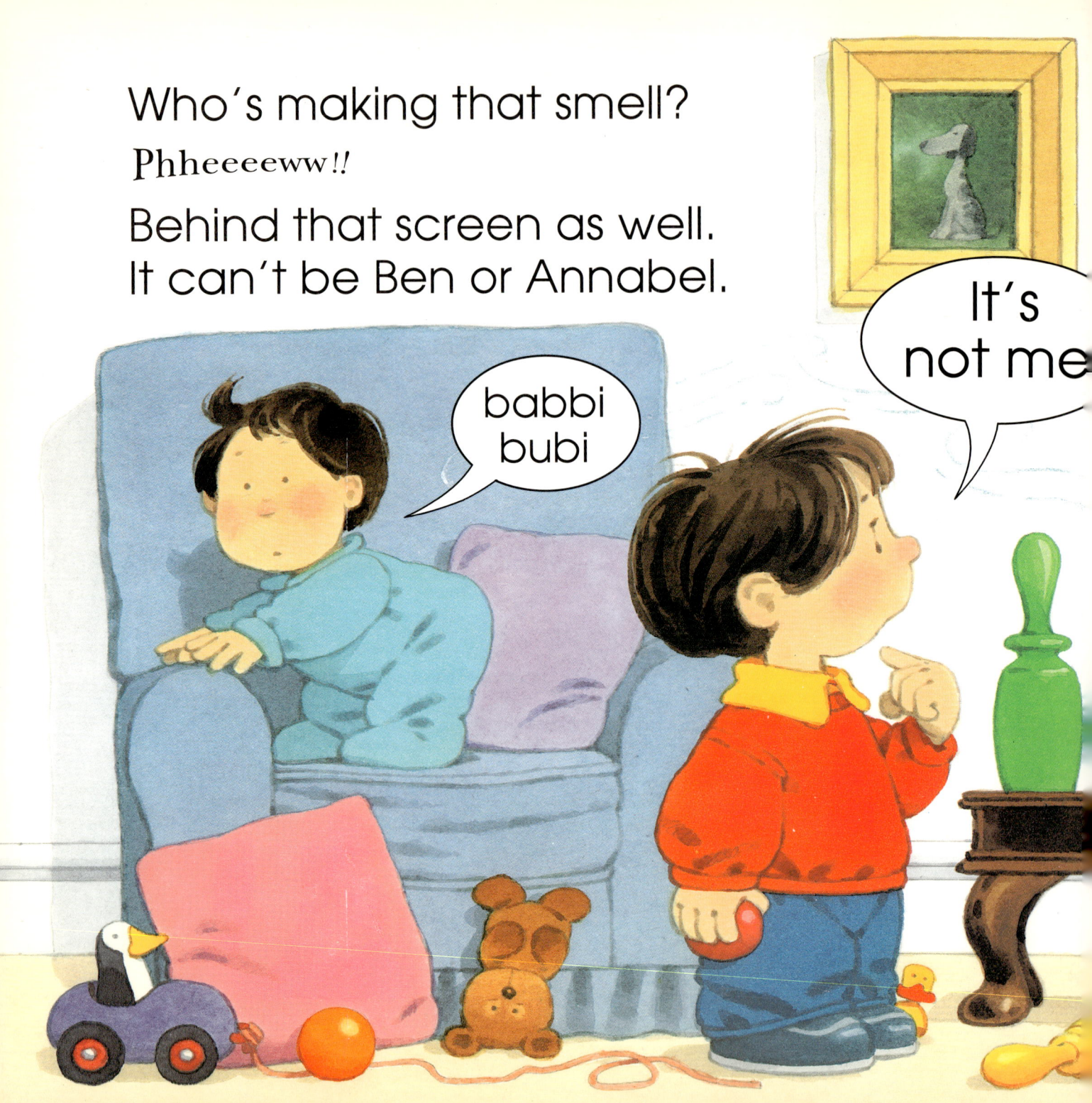

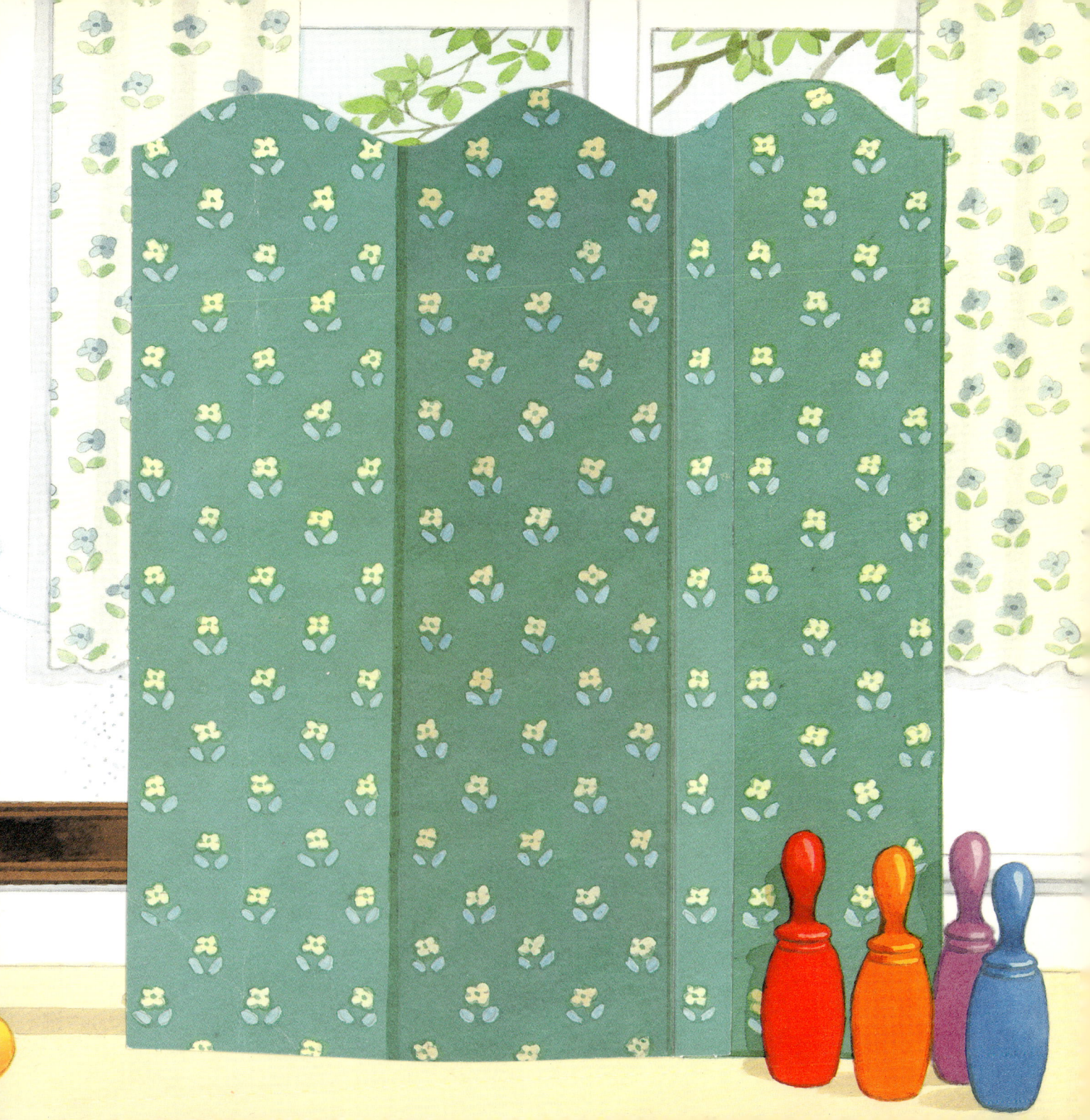

Who's making that smell?
OOooooo₀₀ₒₒₒₒhh!!
It could be caramel.
Is it Ben or Annabel?

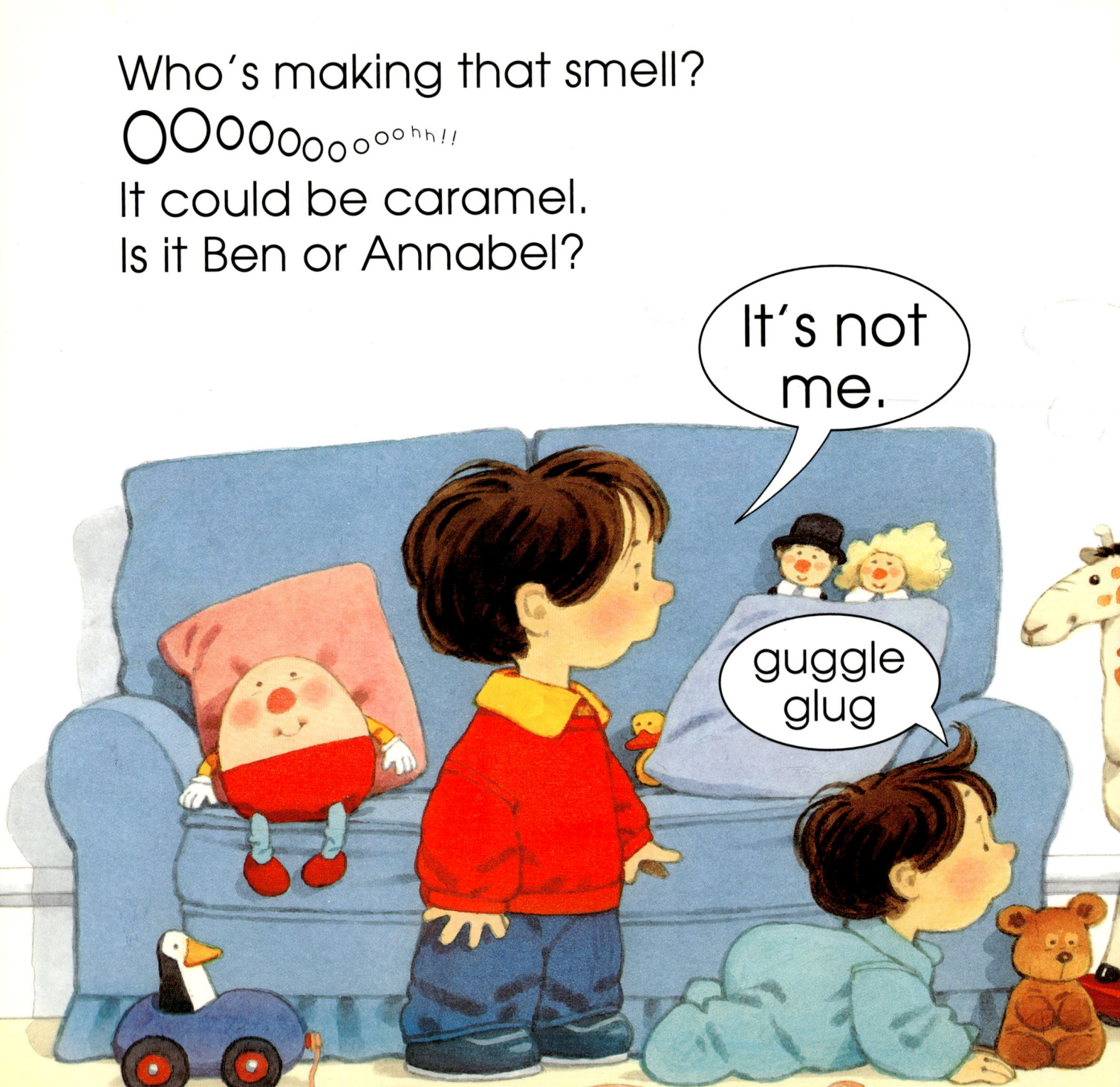

It's not me.

guggle glug

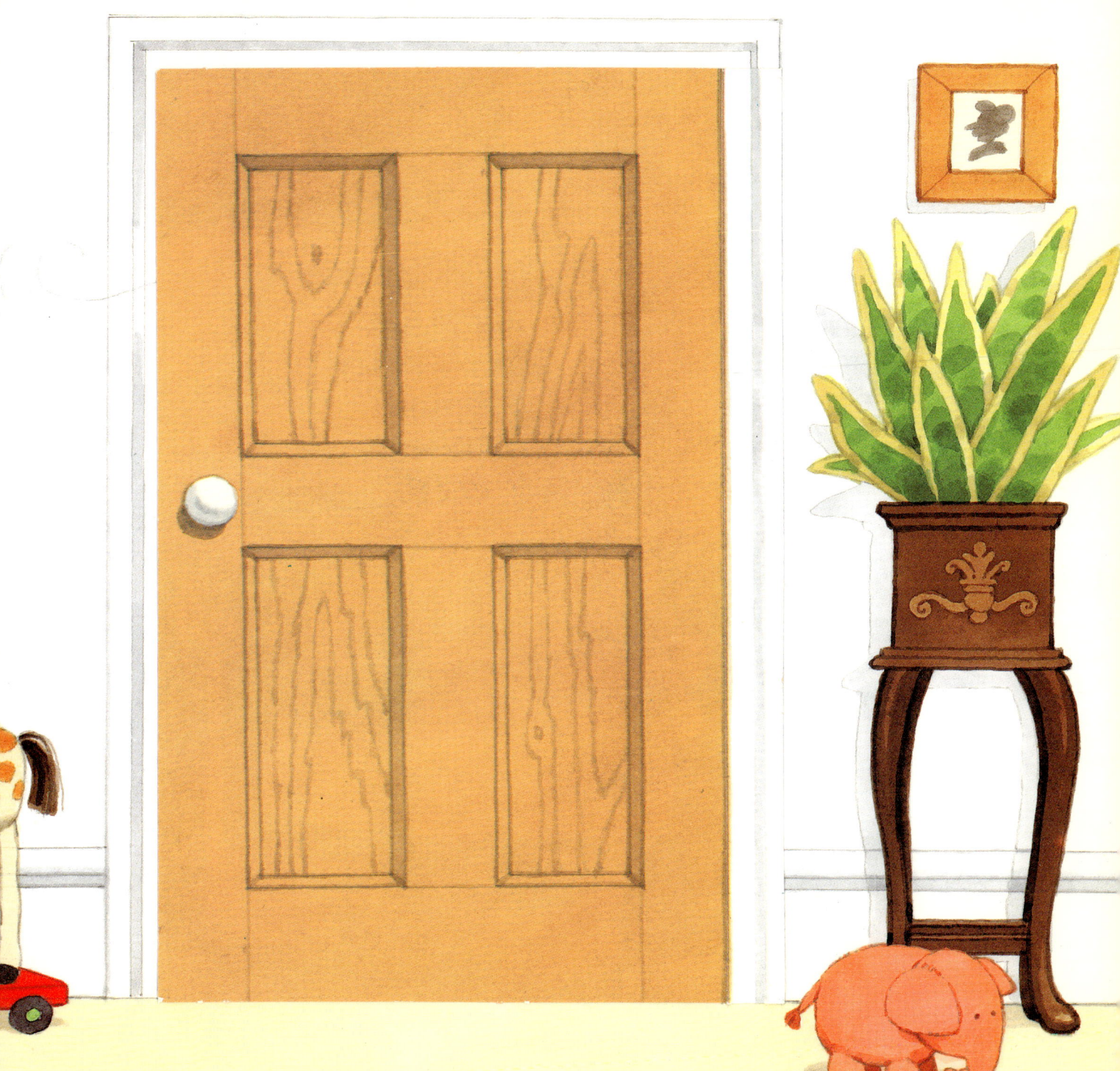

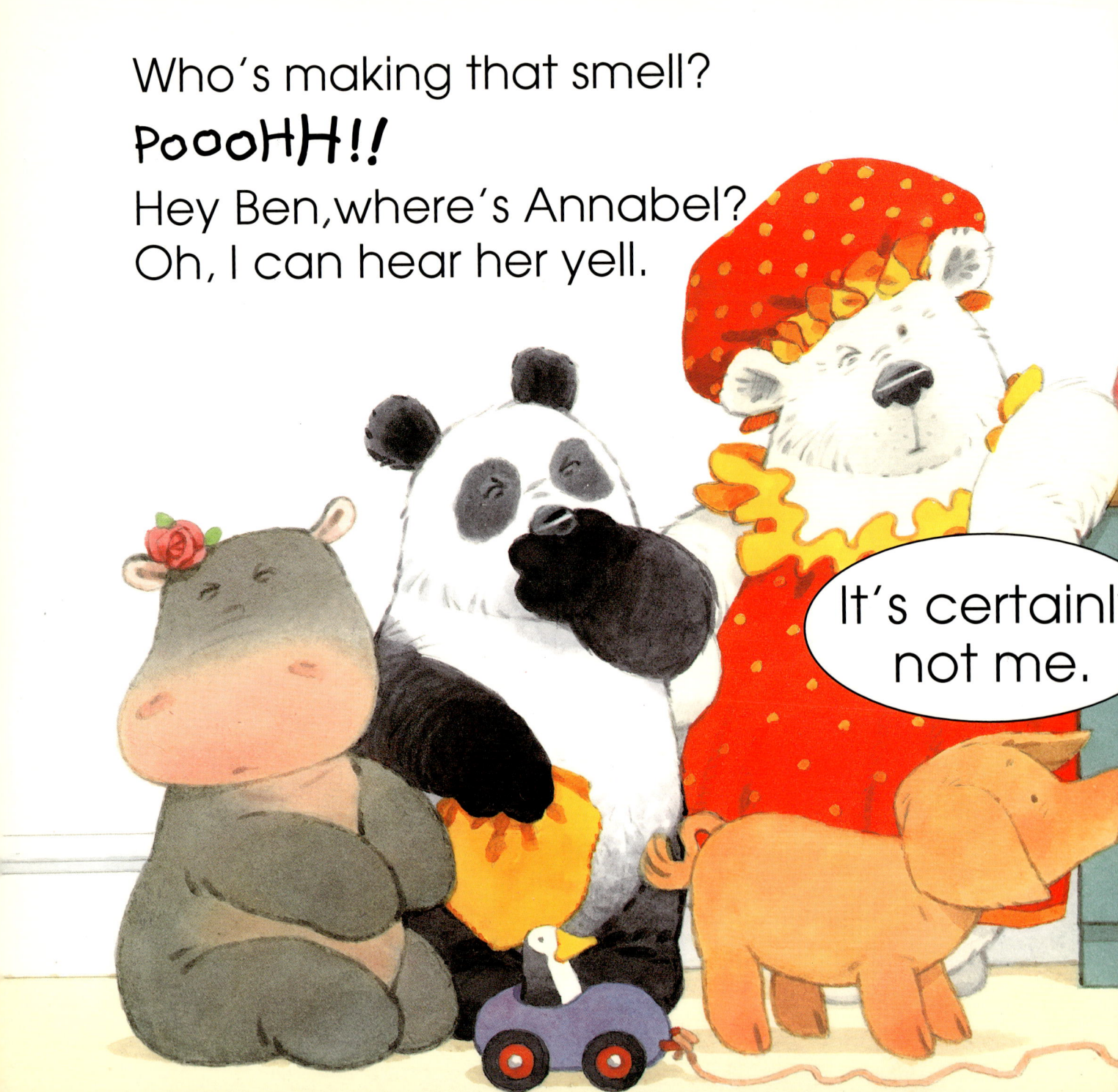

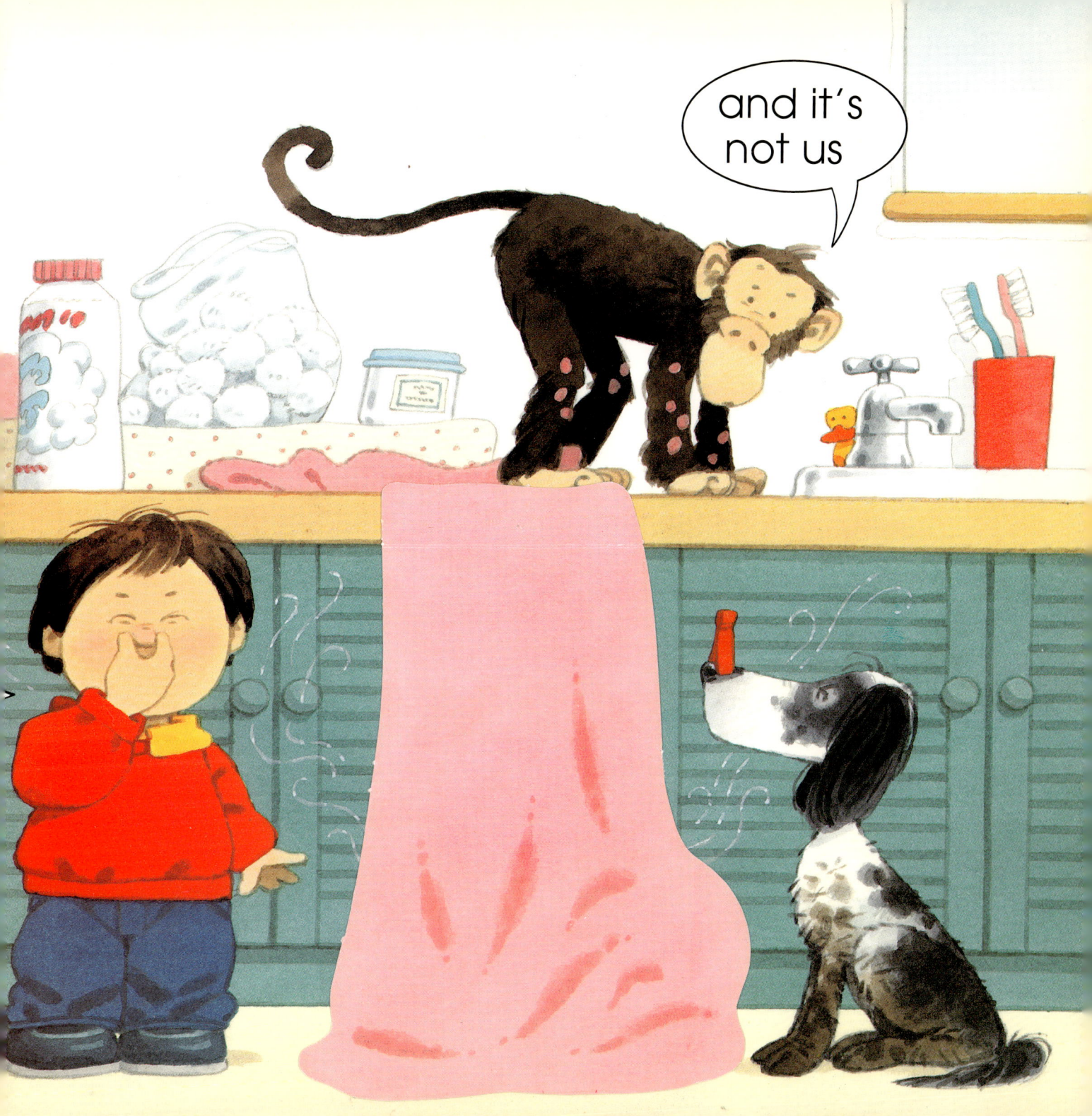

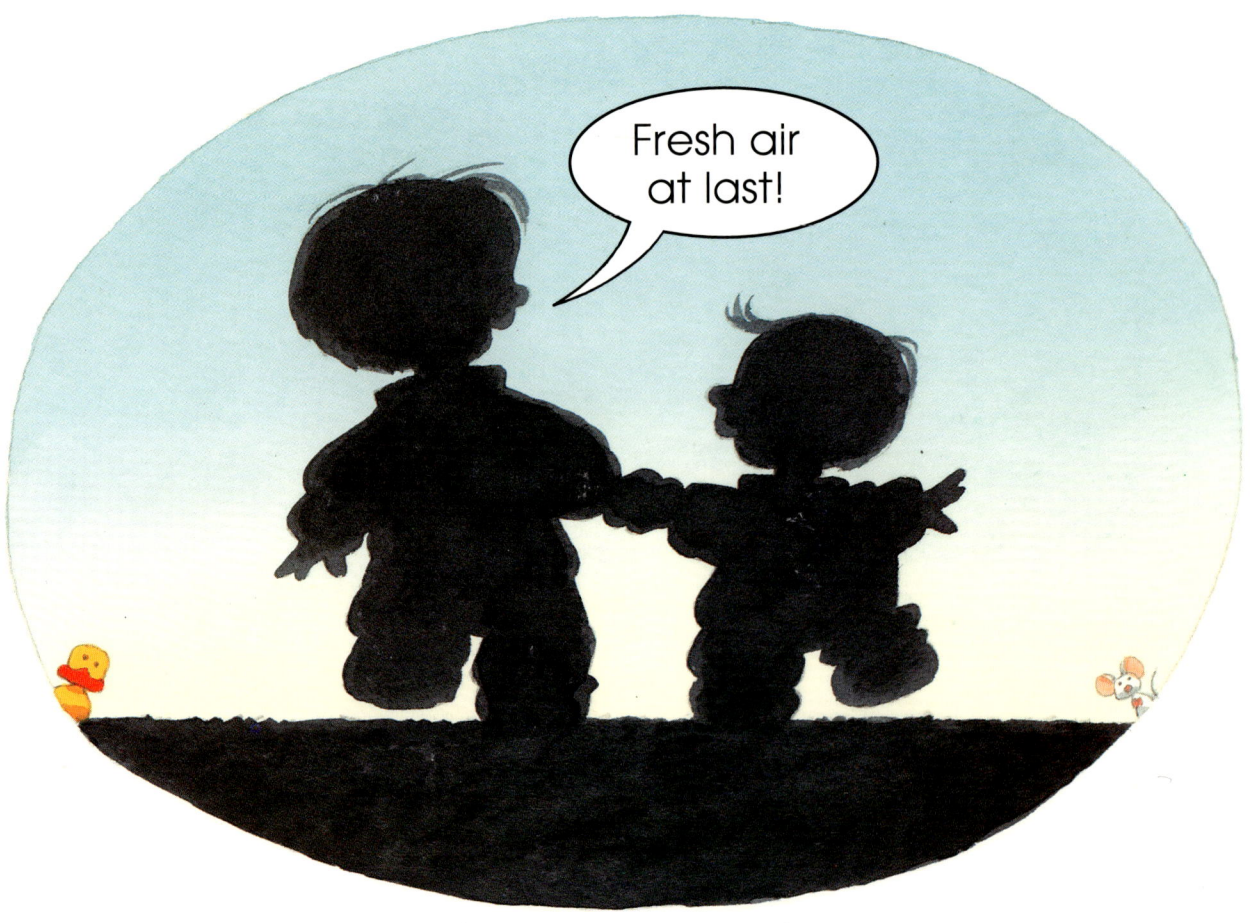

© This Edition: Baby's First Book Club®, Bristol, PA 19007.

Copyright © 1994 Usborne Publishing Ltd. London.
The original titles, "Who's making that noise?" and "Who's making that smell?"
were first published in Great Britain.

All rights reserved. No part of this publication may be reproduced, stored in a retrieval system
or transmitted in any form or by any means, electronic, mechanical, photocopying, recording or otherwise,
without the prior permission from the publisher.

Printed in Singapore
ISBN 1-58048-006-3